The Blood Pressure Solution - Control Your Blood Pressure Naturally

I0411530

Edgar Ortega

+++++++++++++++++++++++++++++++

The Blood Pressure Solution - Control Your Blood Pressure Naturally

Edgar Ortega

ISBN-13: 978-1511594516

ISBN-10: 1511594519

+++++++++++++++++++++++++++++++

Contents

Introduction

Chapter 1: A Silent Epidemic

Chapter 2: The Hidden Dangers of High Blood Pressure

Breaking Down Blood Vessels

Hurting Your Heart

Killing Your Kidneys

Brain Damage

Problems in the Bedroom

Eye Opening Issues

Bad to the Bone

Chapter 3: Understanding Blood Pressure

What Is Blood Pressure?

What Do The Numbers Mean?

How Can We Change Our Blood Pressure?

Chapter 4: Common Causes of High Blood Pressure

Chapter 5: The Healthcare Industry's Answer to High Blood Pressure

Chapter 6: The Blood Pressure Solution: Naturally Lower Your Blood Pressure

Category 1: Dietary Adjustments

Category 2: Smart Supplementation

Category 3: Reducing Body Fat

Category 4: Exercise

Category 5: Stress Reduction

Category 6: Eliminating Toxins

Chapter 7: The Blood Pressure Solution: Implementation Plan

Introduction

On behalf of the entire Primal Health team, I want to thank you for purchasing the Blood Pressure Solution!

This guide is more than just a collection of commonly found advice; instead it is a system that works together to tackle high blood pressure holistically and from many diferent angles. By attacking many of the underlying causes of high blood pressure at once, you will create a synergistic efect that will dramatically elevate your health and help you regain normal blood pressure readings.

There is something else that is diferent about this guide as well.

This guide was built out of necessity.

In 2011 my 65-year-old dad was in bad shape. His weight had slowly but surely crept up the last several years. Also, his energy levels were very low…

and along with that came irritability and mood swings. As so often is the case, my mom intuitively knew that something was up.

My mom had convinced him to visit a free local health fair to get a checkup.

Dad didn't like to go see doctors and she felt like this would be a way to at least have a nurse check his basic vitals. Her hope was that everything was ok, but she could sense that something was amiss with dad's health. That afternoon, as the nurse put the blood pressure cuf on him and began the process of taking his blood pressure reading, she got a strange look in her eyes.

+++++++++++++++++++++++++++++++

7

In fact, she got fustered and started to bark out orders to my parents. Her words to my dad went something like this:

"Sir, you need to go to the emergency room right now. I mean right now…

immediately! Your blood pressure is so high you could have a stroke any minute. Go now!"

My parents knew she wasn't joking but Dad just hated the thought of going to a doctor and having to be put on several diferent high blood pressure medications. He had watched his friend Steve go through this same thing and had witnessed the devastating efect that all these medications had had on Steve. Not only were the side efects of multiple high blood pressure medications making Steve miserable, but the monthly cost was nothing to laugh at either.

So Dad convinced my mom to just take him home and let him try the natural way to lower blood pressure.

Let me be clear: if you are sufering from extremely high blood pressure readings I am not suggesting you avoid your doctor!

However, what I am suggesting is that you give this program a try. It really works and isn't suggesting anything weird or odd. It's hardly controversial, and honestly, it's very efective. The name of the game is to remove the things that increase your blood pressure, and incorporate the things that naturally lower your blood pressure. It's pretty simple, really.

++++++++++++++++++++++++++++++++

8

Naturally, when I found out about my dad's skyrocketing blood pressure results I had to share with him everything I had learned, and how a few simple changes could get his blood pressure under control.

Having firted with high blood pressure myself a year earlier than my dad, and after experimenting with several approaches, I had stumbled across a method of slightly altering my lifestyle, just slightly enough to get my blood pressure back in the normal range.

The information I shared with him worked wonders, and this is not an exaggeration in the least.

Today my dad is 66 yrs. old, works out at the local YMCA every day (sometimes twice a day), and has more energy and vitality that he had when he was in his 40's.

"I probably wouldn´t be

alive. I´ve told Ken several

time: Ken a I look back

in hindsight, you saved

my life".

++++++++++++++++++++++++++++

Now, I don't know if you bought this book because you wanted to yourself, or if you had someone like my mom pushing you to take a serious look at your health, and fnd out what was wrong.

Either way, we are going to begin with the assumption that you have either been recently diagnosed, or feel pretty confdent that you have prehypertension or high blood pressure.

Before I begin teaching you how to naturally lower your blood pressure, I want you to fully realize just how serious having high blood pressure really is.

Unfortunately, most people never fnd out until its too late.

++++++++++++++++++++++++++++

CHAPTER 1

A Silent Epidemic

High blood pressure has been called the 'silent killer'. This is because much of the damage it causes to your cardiovascular system, brain, kidneys, and other organs does not immediately present any noticeable signs such as pain or discomfort. Instead, the insidious nature of high blood pressure works silently to undermine your health with devastating consequences.

Did you know that high blood pressure (hypertension) is indicated as either the primary or contributing cause of death for over 1,000 deaths per day in the United States alone?

Did you know that high blood pressure is the leading cause of stroke?

Did you know that high blood pressure is a major cause of heart attacks?

Research shows us that about 69% of people who have a frst heart attack, 77% who have a frst stroke, and 74% who have congestive heart failure, also have blood pressure.

In the United States, over 31% of the adult population has high blood pressure. That's 1 in 3 adults! That works out to around 78 million people,
++++++++++++++++++++++++++++++++

and the research confrms that only about half of them have their high blood pressure under control.

What's even more alarming is the fact that another 30% of the U.S. population sufers from prehypertension. This means that their elevated blood pressure readings are not yet high enough to make a diagnosis of full-blown hypertension. However, the diagnosis of prehypertension should be taken as a serious warning. Without immediate dietary and lifestyle changes, they will be facing the development of hypertension in the near future.

All told, around 160 million U.S. adults are sufering with a condition that, when uncontrolled, can lead them to having a stroke, heart attack, kidney damage, and even brain damage.

As you can see, not only is high blood pressure a silent killer...but it has also become a silent epidemic.

Resources:

1. n.a. "High Blood Pressure Facts", Centers for Disease Control and Prevention.USA.gov. March 20, 2013. April 23, 2013. http://www.cdc.gov/bloodpressure/facts.htm.

2. n.a. "Heart Disease Facts", Centers for Disease Control and Prevention.USA.gov.March 19, 2013. April 23, 2013.

http://www.cdc.gov/heartdisease/facts.htm.

++++++++++++++++++++++++++++++++

CHAPTER 2

The Hidden Dangers of

High Blood Pressure

Perhaps the most insidious thing about high blood

pressure is that fact that it presents almost no

symptoms that you can readily identify. Instead, it

silently works to undermine your health from the

inside out...often with devastating consequences.

In fact, the list of life-threatening conditions that are directly caused by high blood pressure is stunning.

Breaking Down Blood Vessels

Perhaps the greatest damage that high blood pressure does is to damage the vessels that move the blood around your body. This is a critical transport system that delivers oxygen and nutrients, and takes away carbon dioxide and wastes.

In particular, high blood pressure afects the arteries. These are the vessels that take blood away from the heart to deliver oxygen and nutrition. They are under a higher amount of pressure than that of the veins, which take blood back to the heart.

+++++++++++++++++++++++++++++++

13

Having constantly high pressure causes the cells that make up the inside of your blood vessels to become damaged. They can actually become hardened. You might think at frst that this makes them stronger, but it actually makes them weaker.

The tissue of the blood vessels needs to be elastic so that it can stretch when pressure increases, and go back to its original shape when pressure decreases. But when arteries become hard, they can't expand and contract.

When you consume a lot of high processed foods, and your diet includes foods containing four, sugar, and any of those manufactured 'food-like'

ingredients, all of that 'bad' type of fat in your diet can collect in the hardened areas of the arteries, and eventually cause blockages. Because this system delivers blood to all parts of the body, blockages can cause many of those parts to receive reduced amounts of nutrition and oxygen.

It's important to note that a high fat diet isn't the cause of blockages in your arteries. Rather it is the combination of 'bad' fats, in conjunction with consuming high amounts of processed foods, which results in the killer combination. In fact, recent studies show that a diet with higher fat content, as long as processed foods are removed from the diet, can help bring a person's overall health markers back into normal ranges.

Eventually blockages can lead to heart attacks, a condition where the heart doesn't get enough oxygen and tissue actually dies. You can also become the victim of a stroke, which is bleeding in the brain that has the same result of tissue death.

++++++++++++++++++++++++++++++++

14

When arteries become weak, they can develop aneurysms. These are areas of weak walls in the arteries that bubble out. As they bubble out, they become stretched and unnaturally thin.

Eventually these can burst and can be a cause of stroke. You can also bleed to death internally when an aneurysm bursts, and there are often no symptoms that this is even happening until it is too late to repair the damage.

If all this sounds pretty scary, it should. Heart disease and stroke are the number one killers of both men and women, higher than any cancers or other illnesses. This isn't something to be taken lightly.

Hurting Your Heart

While we've discussed how heart attacks can happen when arteries are damaged, there are some other problems caused by high blood pressure that can afect the heart.

When your heart is constantly under arterial high blood pressure, it has to work harder. This constant wear and tear on the heart can cause it to simply get weak, and wear out.

Even if you don't have a heart attack, you can still sufer from heart failure. As the heart becomes weaker, it's not able to pump nutrients and gases to the tissues, and this begins to afect all systems of the body.

If you have had a heart attack that's damaged your heart, this progression into heart failure can happen even faster. This greatly increases your risk of future heart attacks and heart failure.

++++++++++++++++++++++++++++++++

15

You can also have problems specifcally afecting the arteries that supply blood to your heart. These are called coronary arteries. They're specialized in that they deliver blood to and from your heart in order to provide it with oxygen and nutrients.

If they become hardened or blocked, they can cause your heart to perform at a lower rate, and even cause a heart attack. They can also cause you to have an irregular heartbeat or chest pain.

Normally your heart is about the size of your fst, but when you have high blood pressure you can sufer from an enlarged heart on one side. The left side of your heart is responsible for delivering blood to the rest of the body.

When you have high blood pressure, this side can get harder and larger, as well. An enlarged heart is not as efcient as a heart that's the normal size for your body. This can increase your risk of a heart attack and heart disease.

Killing Your Kidneys

Your kidneys are also greatly afected by having high blood pressure. Many people don't know that these organs help to regulate your blood pressure by decreasing or increasing the fuid in your blood.

When you have high blood pressure, your kidneys can actually develop scars. Within your kidneys are millions of tiny blood vessels that become damaged when they're exposed to constant high pressure.

+++++++++++++++++++++++++++++++

16

As they become scarred, they're less able to do their job of fltering blood. This can cause your body to not be unable to flter waste properly, and can lead to kidney disease.

You can also have an aneurysm in the blood vessels of your kidneys. This type of aneurysm is very deadly due to the amount of blood that travels through your kidneys. Because your entire blood supply passes through them, you could die from massive internal bleeding.

Finally, you may develop kidney failure. Kidney failure is the inability of your kidneys to flter waste either because of damage to the large or the small arteries that deliver blood to them.

When this happens you may have a buildup of toxins, as well as swelling, due to an increased amount of bodily fuids. Over time you may require dialysis. This is a necessary procedure that involves removing the blood from your blood, and then fltering it through a machine, which is then sent back to the body.

Ultimately, having kidney failure may result in the need for having a kidney transplant. However, the list for this is very long, and the poorer your overall health is, the less likely you are to get an organ transplant.

Brain Damage

High blood pressure is also very bad for the brain. As we already discussed, high blood pressure puts you at increased risk of stroke. The efects of a stroke can include paralysis, memory loss, and even death.

+++++++++++++++++++++++++++++++

17

However, there are other problems associated with high blood pressure. For example, people with high blood pressure are at a greater risk for dementia.

This can come as a result of not having enough oxygen being delivered to the brain.

You can also have impairment to your brain that keeps you from being able to process information. The earlier in life that you begin to experience high blood pressure, the greater the damage will become as you age.

Problems in the Bedroom

One of the most common causes of erectile dysfunction in men is high blood pressure. High blood pressure afects all the blood vessels in the body and can decrease fow to the penis.

But if you are a woman, don't think that you're of the hook. Women also rely on strong blood fow to the vaginal area for sexual arousal and satisfac-tion. So both men and women should be aware of this issue so that both sexes are able to identify and prevent any problems of this nature.

In fact, treating high blood pressure often eliminates the need to take drugs, such as Viagra, for sexual dysfunction. Your best bet for good sexual health is maintaining good heart health.

Difculty sleeping is another factor to consider. Studies note that high blood pressure and sleep apnea go hand in hand. Sleep apnea keeps you from getting enough sleep, and actually puts you at risk for heart disease and other problems.

++++++++++++++++++++++++++++++++

18

Eye Opening Issues

Your eyes are also very sensitive to changes in your blood pressure. The blood vessels of the eyes are very small and fragile, and are particularly vulnerable to being damaged as a result of having high blood pressure.

When the retina is not correctly supplied with blood, it can become damaged. You can have blurred vision, or even a complete loss of vision, when blood pressure goes unchecked.

If you also have the secondary condition of diabetes, you're particularly at risk for this type of problem. Diabetes and high blood pressure greatly increase your risk of eye disease and loss of sight.

Additionally, you could face is blockage in the blood vessels leading to your optic nerve. This, too, can lead to permanent blurred vision, and even blind-ness. So it's critical that you pay attention to your blood pressure to maintain good vision.

Finally, ongoing high blood pressure can cause a buildup of fuid in your eye.

The excess pressure this creates can cause damage and scarring inside the eye, which can lead to permanent vision deterioration.

Bad to the Bone

You might be surprised to know that you can even sufer from bone loss as a result of problems with your blood pressure. People with high blood pressure lose more calcium than those who have normal blood pressure.

++++++++++++++++++++++++++++++

19

As calcium leaves the bones and enters the bloodstream, bones can be left weak and brittle. This increases your risk for both osteoporosis, as well as a greater risk of broken bones due to injury. In fact, most hip fractures in seniors are actually a result of bone disease.

While men can sufer from osteoporosis, women are generally more at risk after menopause. It is important to keep track of your blood pressure, and take corrective action whenever necessary.

Resources

1.Mayo Clinic staf."High blood pressure dangers: Hypertension's efects on your body". High blood pressure (hypertension). Mayo Clinic. Mayo Foundation for

Medical Education and Research. Jan. 21, 2011. April 23, 2013.

http://www.mayoclinic.com/health/highblood-pressure/HI00062

2. n.a, "High Blood Pressure Damages the Brain in Early Middle Age". UC Davis Health System. October 31, 2012.

April 23. 2013. http://www.ucdmc.ucdavis.edu/publish/news/newsroom/7118

+++++++++++++++++++++++++++++++

20

CHAPTER 3

Understanding Blood

Pressure

Before you can fx something, you have to

understand how it works. Blood pressure doesn't

have to be a mystery. In fact, solving the riddle of

high blood pressure is really more of a mechanical problem than anything else. In the following

chapter I'll explain what blood pressure is, and

show you the seven blood press levers that we can

manipulate in order to naturally control our blood

pressure.

Follow along, and you'll see what I mean....

What Is Blood Pressure?

With all the numbers you have to keep track of, you may be a bit confused about the biological importance of maintaining proper blood pressure levels, and what exactly those numbers represent. Quite literally, the numbers associated with your blood pressure readings indicates the exact amount of pressure being exerted on the walls of your blood vessels, as your blood fows throughout your body, at any given time.

+++++++++++++++++++++++++++++++++

Your blood vessels are basically a set of interconnected tubes, of which you have two types. The frst are your arteries, which carry oxygen rich blood from the heart to your organs and cells. The second are your veins, responsible for carrying your blood back to your heart again.

When we talk about blood pressure, we are referring to the amount of force created as your blood is rushing through your arteries. It is important to know how much pressure is being created, as this determines how to properly regulate the force required to keep your arteries open. The process works much like the way water runs through a garden hose. The amount of force created by the water as it fows through the hose determines whether or not the hose stays open and taut.

If your blood pressure is too low, blood can't be transported properly to all the cells of your body. If it's too high, you're at risk for heart disease and even stroke. This is why it's important to keep your blood pressure within the normal range to maintain optimum health.

What Do The Numbers Mean?

Blood Pressure Category Systolic Diastolic

   mm Hg (upper #) mm Hg (lower #)

Normal less than 120 and less than 80

Prehypertension 120-139 or 80-89

High Blood Pressure Stage 1 (Hypertension) 140-159 or 90-99

High Blood Pressure Stage 2 (Hypertension) 160 or higher or 100 or higher Hypertensive Crisis

(Emergency Care Needed)

Higher than 180 or Higher than 110

              +++++++++++++++++++++++++++++++

When your heart is at rest, your blood pressure is lower. This is the diastolic pressure, represented by the bottom number of your blood pressure reading. Ideally, you want this number to be close to 80.

As your heart begins actively pumping, this creates more pressure on the walls of your blood vessels. The amount indicates your systolic pressure, which is represented by the top number of your blood pressure reading.

You want this to be close to 120.

Again, these numbers are the actual measurements of pressure being applied to the blood vessel walls. Your healthcare provider can take your blood pressure using a special cuf and instrument called a sphygmoma-nometer. You can also check your own blood pressure using digital machines that are often located in your local pharmacy, or even purchase one for yourself to keep at home.

Having high blood pressure one time isn't a big problem. Stress, infections, and activity can cause changes in blood pressure. But taking consistent readings when you're at rest will give you a picture of your overall blood pressure, and if it's consistently high, you need to pay attention.

The bottom number is the one you need to pay the most attention to. It's not as likely to fuctuate with other changes in the body. But when the bottom number is high you're more at risk for problems.

++++++++++++++++++++++++++++++

23

How Can We Change Our Blood Pressure?

Going back to the example of a garden hose, let's think about what factors could have an impact on the pressure inside the hose as water is fowing through it. This will give us a clue as to how we plan to control your blood pressure. A garden hose is simply a fexible tube, much like a blood vessel.

In our example, let's assume we have a pump on the end of the garden hose that is going to rhythmically push the water through the hose, just like your heart pushes blood through your blood vessels.

THE IDENTIFIABLE VARIABLES THAT HAVE AN IMPACT ON THE

PRESSURE being put on the interior walls of the garden hose are: 1. The amount of water fowing inside the hose. The more water that's fowing, the higher the pressure.

2. The viscosity of the water. This means how freely it fows due to its thickness or

thinness.

3. The force of the pump pushing the water through the hose 4. The rate at which the pump cycles and pushes water through the hose

5. The fexibility of the hose walls to expand, thereby creating more interior space inside the hose

6. The external pressure being applied to the outside walls of the hose

7. Any blockages or deposits inside the hose that reduce its interior space.

++++++++++++++++++++++++++++++

24

Believe it or not, these are the same seven variables that we can begin to manipulate within our own bodies through the proper use of diet, exercise, certain natural supplements, and even some simple lifestyle changes.

Let me restate these same seven variables in terms that apply to blood pressure, which I call the Seven Blood Pressure Levers.

++++++++++++++++++++++++++++++

25

The Seven Blood Pressure Levers:

• The amount of blood inside our blood vessels

• The viscosity of our blood (how thin or thick it is impacts how easily it fows)

• The strength of our heart (our pump)

• The rate of our heartbeat

• The fexibility, or ability for our blood vessels to relax and be less tense • The reduction in external pressure on our blood vessels via weight loss • The reduction of any blockages within or blood vessels These seven variables are the key to knowing the 'What' of lowering your blood pressure. In fact, these same seven variables are exactly the same seven methods that modern medicine focuses on with its medicines.

However, prescription medication can often come with devastating and unpleasant side efects. But we will cover more on that later.

Resources:

1. n.a. "High Blood Pressure" MedlinePlus, U.S. National Library of Medicine, NIH.Updated 22 April 2013. April 23, 2013. http://www.nlm.nih.gov/medlineplus/highbloodpressure.html 2. n.a. "What is High Blood Pressure?" American Heart Association. Mar 1, 2013. April 23, 2013.

http://www.heart.org/HEARTORG/Conditions/HighBloodPressure/AboutHighBloodPi is-HighBlood-Pressure_UCM_301759_Article.jsp

3. George L. Bakris, MD. "High Blood Pressure". The Merck Manual, Home Health Handbook.Merck Sharp &

Dohme Corp, Merck & Co., Inc. March 2013. April 23, 2013.

http://www.merckmanuals.com/home/heart_and_blood_vessel_disorders/high_blood_]

+++++++++++++++++++++++++++++++

CHAPTER 4

Common Causes Of High

Blood Pressure

Your blood pressure can fluctuate to some degree,

even when you just walk into the doctor's ofce,

especially if you're nervous. But it won't change too

much unless you've been sufering from one of the

conditions that is highly correlated to having high

blood pressure.

Also, your blood pressure might naturally begin to

increase as you age. Because your blood vessels

aren't as fexible when you're older, they tend to become more rigid.

Below are some other common factors:

• Overweight individuals have more instances of hypertension.

• Changing hormones can afect your blood pressure levels.

• Genetics play a role in whether or not you have hypertension.

• Stress and anxiety can cause spikes in your blood pressure.

• Diabetics experience more instances of high blood pressure.

• Too much salt (sodium) is a contributing factor to high blood pressure readings.

• The shape of your blood vessels will help or hurt your blood pressure.

++++++++++++++++++++++++++++++

• If your kidneys are in bad shape, this can cause high blood pressure.

• Smokers receive a diagnosis of hypertension more often than non-smokers.

• Overloading on alcohol can cause high blood pressure readings.

• A potassium defciency or vitamin D defciency can contribute to hypertension.

• African Americans tend to have a higher risk of hypertension.

The medical community classifes high blood pressure, or hypertension, into two broad categories - Primary and Secondary Hypertension.

Secondary hypertension is when high blood pressure levels are caused by a specifc medical condition, like kidney disease.

Primary hypertension is diagnosed when doctors are unable to determine a specifc medical condition that could be to blame for your high blood pressure. This is the case in almost 90-95% of the people diagnosed with high blood pressure.

However, this doesn't mean that you can't do anything about your high blood pressure.

Instead, what it points to is something I call Lifestyle Induced High Blood Pressure.

This is simply a case of high blood pressure that was brought about due solely to poor lifestyle choices. While this might make you feel a little down at frst, this is actually great news!

+++++++++++++++++++++++++++++++

This means that you are in complete control of your blood pressure. Having high blood pressure came as a result of specifc choices you've made along the way. But now you will understand how to make better choices, and how those choices will allow you to achieve better results. By appropriately modifying your lifestyle, you can get rid of high blood pressure, and avoid all the negative health issues that come with it.

Resources:

1. NewsUSA. "Black men continue to lead in hypertension statistics".stltoday.com. March 26, 2013. April 23, 1013.

http://www.stltoday.com/lifestyles/healthmed-ft/golden-age/black-men-continue-to-lead-in-hypertension-statistics/article_99804a15-b5e8-5456-a9b2-35a598263397.html

2. n.a. "Too much salt may damage blood vessels and lead to high blood pressure". American Heart Association.

June 18, 2012. April 23, 2013. http://newsroom.heart.org/news/too-much-salt-may-damage-blood-235113

+++++++++++++++++++++++++++++++

CHAPTER 5

The Healthcare Industry's

Answer To High Blood

Pressure

So let's say you were recently diagnosed with high

blood pressure. For most people this usually

occurs during a routine ofce visit with your

family doctor, or like my dad, maybe you visited

a local health fair and found out that your blood

pressure was too high.

As I mentioned before, you should always monitor your blood pressure readings for a period of a

week or so to determine the average of your blood pressure readings.

A single high reading isn't usually a cause for alarm unless it is dangerously high and requires immediate medical attention.

But let's say you monitored your blood pressure for a few days and found that you were indeed reading high.

During your visit to your doctor you were probably told to stop eating salt, exercise more, and get on a few specifc medications.

++++++++++++++++++++++++++++++++

30

Let me be clear…some people need to be on prescription drugs to control their high blood pressure. However, many people do not and can control their high blood pressure without the need for prescription drugs, which are not only expensive but often come with unpleasant side efects.

A treatment plan will often include an ACE inhibitor and a beta-blocker along with other medication that are adjusted to the individual patient's needs.

Here is a list of the most common high blood pressure medications, tradi-tionally prescribed by the medical community:

ACE Inhibitors

How they work: This type of drug blocks the creation of a specifc chemical in your body that causes your blood vessels to constrict. The result is that without this chemical, your blood vessels relax and allow blood to fow more easily than before.

Side efects include: hypotension, cough, headache, dizziness, fatigue, nausea, and renal impairment.

Alpha Blockers

How They Work: Alpha-blockers also help with relaxing the blood vessels so that blood can fow more easily.

Side efects include: dizziness from rapid decreases in blood pressure, headache, pounding heartbeat, nausea, weakness, and weight gain.

++++++++++++++++++++++++++++++++

31

Beta Blockers

How They Work: Beta-blockers work by blocking naturally occurring epinephrine, also known as adrenaline. This has the efect of keeping your heart rate slower and pumping with less force, thereby pushing less blood through your system and lowering blood pressure.

Side efects include: fatigue, cold hands, headache, upset stomach, constipa-tion, diarrhea, and dizziness.

Diuretics

How They Work: Diuretics work by causing your body to get rid of water.

This has two efects that are important to lowering blood pressure. First it reduces the volume of blood in your blood vessels (blood is made up of about 50% water), which creates less pressure inside your blood vessels.

Second, as the fuid is being released out of your body it takes with it much of the salt, as well. This also helps to reduce blood pressure.

Side efects: Unfortunately a diuretic cannot distinguish between good minerals in your bodily fuid so it also fushes out many of the benefcial minerals such as potassium. Other side efects include weakness, muscle cramps due to fushing potassium out of your system, dizziness, blurred vision, headache, fever, sore throat, ringing in ears, skin rash, nausea.

Vasodilators

How They Work: Vasodilators work by opening up or dilating your blood vessels, creating more interior room for proper blood fow. This lowers the pressure inside the blood vessel due to the extra room created when the blood vessel expands.

+++++++++++++++++++++++++++++++++

32

Side efects include: rapid heartbeat, headaches, dizziness, nausea, vomit-ing, bloating, sore throat, joint pain, swollen feet or legs, fushing, swollen lymph nodes, fever, skin blisters, or itching.

As you have probably realized, these medications try to manipulate all seven of the exact same variables that we identifed in the frst part of this book.

These are the very same variables that we can all manipulate via natural methods, and change our blood pressure for the better. Here they are again for your review:

The Seven Blood Pressure Levers:

• The amount of blood inside our blood vessels

• The viscosity of our blood (how thin or thick it is impacts how easily it fows)

• The strength of our heart (our pump)

• The rate of our heartbeat

• The fexibility, or ability for our blood vessels to relax and be less tense • The reduction in external pressure on our blood vessels via weight loss • The reduction of any blockages within or blood vessels The next question you should be asking yourself is this:

If the medical community knows that it is 100% possible to naturally lower blood pressure without medications that carry such devastating side efects, why do they continue to prescribe these medications?

+++++++++++++++++++++++++++++++++

33

There can only be a few possible answers to that question, but the bottom line is:

1. Ignorance: they simply don't know you can lower your blood pressure naturally.

2. Self-Interest: they want you to be on medication and dependent upon their prescriptions.

3. Lack of Faith: they simply don't believe that you have the ability to change your diet and behavior. So they make the choice for you - by prescribing drugs to you that come with serious side efects, which may work as a short-term solution. But in reality, this doesn't address the root cause of your high blood pressure at all!

Wouldn't it be healthier and better for their patients to lower their blood pressure naturally?

YES!

Why deal with those side efects when you can just as easily, and far less expensively, lower your blood pressure with some simple dietary and lifestyle changes?

That is exactly what I am about to teach you how to do!

++++++++++++++++++++++++++++++++

34

Warning: Don't Stop Your Prescriptions Without

Talking To Your Doctor

Again I want to be very clear here that I am not recommending you stop taking any blood pressure medication that you are currently taking. Instead I suggest you talk to your doctor about your desire to lower your blood pressure naturally. Ask him to look over your plan, and help you transition into coming of of your blood pressure drugs in a way that does not harm your health.

However, if you aren't on any of these drugs yet, then I want to encourage you to keep reading. With the information I am about to share, you will fnally have the knowledge necessary to control your high blood pressure using natural cures.

Resources:

1. n.a. "AntiHypertensive Drugs". Baylor Healthcare System. News-Medical.Net. April 23, 2013. April 23, 2013.

http://www.news-medical.net/admin/health/AntiHypertensive-Drugs.aspx 2. George L. Bakris, MD. "High Blood Pressure". The Merck Manual, Home Health Handbook.Merck Sharp & Dohme Corp, Merck & Co., Inc. March 2013. April 23, 2013.

http://www.merckmanuals.com/home/heart_and_blood_vessel_disorders/high_blood_

++++++++++++++++++++++++++++++++

35

CHAPTER 6

The Blood Pressure

Solution: Naturally Lower

Your Blood Pressure!

The Blood Pressure Solution Program is based on the idea that blood pressure is something that can be controlled naturally through smart changes to diet and lifestyle.

To that end, we will be tackling your high blood pressure on many fronts…

all proven to positively improve a person's blood pressure readings.

Remember, these adjustments all work together as a synergistic system, so the more of them you implement…the greater the efect.

One of the interesting things you will start to realize as you begin to implement the strategies in this program is how interrelated the causes and cures to high blood pressure really are.

For example, as you begin to modify your diet by reducing certain nutrients and adding others in, you will most likely start to also lose weight. The reduction of weight will help you lower blood pressure by taking pressure of the outside walls of your blood vessels.

+++++++++++++++++++++++++++++++

36

The reduction of sodium will also cause you to release extra water that is being held in your body. This will reduce the volume of blood in your body as well, which will also help lower your blood pressure. As you begin to eat smarter and exercise more, you will also start to repair the damage to your blood vessels, lowering your blood pressure even more.

There will be many such examples as you begin working through the program. The key point I want to make here is that the changes you will be implementing should be viewed as much more than just individual changes.

Instead they are interconnected and synergistic. They work with each other to provide much more beneft than you would receive if implementing each change on its own.

In order to understand how this program works, let's take one more look at the Seven Blood Pressure Levers:

The Seven Blood Pressure Levers:

• The amount of blood inside our blood vessels

• The viscosity of our blood (how thin or thick it is impacts how easily it fows)

• The strength of our heart (our pump)

• The rate of our heartbeat

• The fexibility, or ability for our blood vessels to relax and be less tense • The reduction in external pressure on our blood vessels via weight loss • The reduction of any blockages within or blood vessels ++++++++++++++++++++++++++++++++

37

In order to change the Seven Blood Pressure Levers, we will be teaching you how to make small but powerful tweaks to your diet and lifestyle in the following six broad categories:

REMEMBER:

These are the same seven levers that the medical community tries to manipulate as well, however they do it with drugs that have many unwanted side efects. We will be modifying these levers the natural way and will be getting excellent results…with very little, if any side efects.

++++++++++++++++++++++++++++++

38

Category 1: Dietary Adjustments

In this section I'll show you how to adjust your diet

so that you eliminate foods that contribute to high

blood pressure, and add in foods that are known

to reduce blood pressure. These foods were cho—

sen because of the special minerals and nutrients

they provide that have been proven to lower blood

pressure.

When I was diagnosed with prehypertension and

the doctor recommended that I start a low dose of high blood pressure medication, I started asking questions about how I could lower my blood pressure naturally. I had always had an aversion to taking medication, and it just made sense to me that if I changed the way I had been treating my body, that my body might have the ability to heal itself.

One of the frst things I did was alter my diet. Within a very short period of time my blood pressure was back within normal ranges. Without a doubt this should be your frst plan of action, as well. Dietary modifcations bring about the biggest changes in blood pressure.

The diet I'm about to teach to you emphasizes foods that are rich in potassium, magnesium and calcium…all minerals that are critical to how your body regulates blood pressure. Most individuals with hypertension usually have either a defciency or an imbalance of these minerals, which are an important part of your diet.

++++++++++++++++++++++++++++++++

39

If you remember the story of how my dad dramatically lowered his blood pressure, then you may remember that one of the frst things he changed was his diet. I shared with him what I had learned, and how by altering my diet I was able to achieve much better health and lowered my blood pressure.

As he began to implement the program I am about to share with you, something amazing started to happen.

First, his blood pressure started to normalize.

Second, he began to lose weight...and a lot of it!

As of this writing dad has lost over 80 lbs. of fat from his body, and at the young age of 66 he is bouncing around like a guy in his late 20's. It's been a lot of fun to watch, and it all started with some simple dietary changes.

The diet I recommend to quickly and dramatically lower your blood pressure is one that is based on the latest research into how our ancient ancestors ate.

Simply put, this diet brings 'real foods' back into the primary focus, and eliminates foods that are heavily processed and full of chemicals, which are harmful for your metabolism and your immune system.

Before we get to the diet that I recommend, I have to talk about the number one item you will need to cut back on immediately...and that is sodium.

However, this topic is not as black and white as you might assume. Let me explain...

+++++++++++++++++++++++++++++++

40

The Sodium Dilemma

Primary on this list of nutrients that you will want to limit is sodium, which most people will relate to common table salt. I remember growing up and watching the other men in my family gather around the kitchen table and begin preparing their plates of food. What was the number one thing almost all of them did? Yes you probably guessed it! They grabbed the saltshaker and applied very generous helpings of salt to almost everything on the plate.

When you couple this common ritual with the fact that almost all processed food is saturated with sodium for its food preservation benefts, you will quickly see how we have become a culture that chronically over consumes sodium.

How Does Sodium Raise Blood Pressure?

If you are like me, you like to know why things work the way they do. Understanding how sodium causes your blood pressure to rise is actually quite helpful and something most people don't fully understand. Think back to our discussion about the Seven Blood Pressure Levers, and you'll remember that the volume of blood fowing through your arteries will impact your blood pressure readings. The more fuid (blood) fowing through the hose (your arteries) the greater the pressure will be. This is a simple law of physics. Well, it turns out that when you consume sodium, another substance inside your body is highly attracted to the sodium. Wherever there is sodium in your body, water is sure to follow. This is why when you eat too many salty foods you start to feel bloated. Sodium makes your body retain water. The impact on your blood pressure is almost immediate as more water in your system also means that the volume of blood in your arteries will also rise. Remember, blood is over 50% water.

+++++++++++++++++++++++++++++++

41

Should I Eliminate Sodium From My Diet?

When you begin to learn about the negative impact that sodium has on your blood pressure, a natural response will be to want to eliminate sodium from your diet altogether. However, this would be a grave mistake. We actually need sodium for our bodies to survive. A certain level of sodium in our body is required for proper cellular communication, which allows for proper muscle contraction, and helps to regulate bodily fuids. The key is to get your sodium intake under control and into healthy ranges, but not to eliminate it entirely.

Sodium Recommendations

The recommended daily amount of sodium intake is no more than 2.3

grams of sodium per day for a healthy adult under age 51. If you have high blood pressure the recommendation is to keep your sodium intake to less than 1.5 grams per day. This is roughly 1/2 teaspoon of sodium per day. Not much, but just enough to provide your body with all the sodium it needs.

Sea Salt: A Healthier Alternative?

While most people think of table salt when they think about sodium, there is actually a diferent kind of salt that is growing in popularity. Allowing seawater to evaporate produces what's called sea salt, a naturally occurring salt. Unlike table salt, which is highly processed and has all the trace minerals removed from it, sea salt preserves the other minerals in it, such as potassium and magnesium, which have been shown to be very benefcial to people with high blood pressure. While the actual amount of sodium in each teaspoon of sea salt is very similar to table salt, there are some manufac-

+++++++++++++++++++++++++++++++

turers of sea salt that claim to have perfected an evaporative process that yields sea salt that has 57% less sodium than table salt. In my opinion, this deserves exploring as an alternative to the overly processed table salt.

Blunting Sodium's Impact With Potassium

Although there will be much more information on potassium in the bonus report "99 Foods That Naturally Lower Blood Pressure", I wanted to mention here that potassium seems to have the ability to counteract some of the efects of sodium in your body. That is why most doctors recommend that you increase the amount of potassium in your diet.

Now that we've covered the important topic of sodium consumption, let's dive back into the diet that I recommend to help with your eforts to lower blood pressure.

Eating To Live

As I began researching ways to naturally lower my own blood pressure, I began to notice a common theme.

The vitamins, minerals, and other nutrient based solutions were most readily accessible through either real foods or in some cases supplements.

When I say real foods, I am talking about foods that have a single ingredient such as a banana, raisins, grapes, spinach, etc.

Nowhere in the research was any processed foods recommended.

43

This realization was a profound moment for me. Essentially I had stumbled upon a basic concept that had eluded me for years.

The more I researched and understood the damaging impact that manufactured foods had on our bodies, the more I started to adopt a very simple way of eating. This style of eating predates the modern era and instead of providing your body with a bewildering array of chemical additives, instead supplies your body with the foods it has thrived on for millennia. Just simple, natural, real food is all your body needs.

Simply put, WE HAVE TWO OPTIONS REGARDING THE TYPES OF

FOOD that we can put into our bodies:

1. Manufactured Foods: these are foods that have been heavily processed in a factory and cannot be found in nature.

They have typically had most or all of their natural nutrients removed, and then flled with chemical additives to provide some taste. Chemical preservatives are also typically added to extend their shelf life. Great examples of these types of foods are pasta, bread, candy, hot dogs, *etc.*

2. Natural (or Whole) Foods: These foods are made up of just one ingredient and typically are either an animal product, or something that grew from the ground. Examples include

sweet potatoes, vegetables, beef, chicken, fsh, *etc.*

44

A Macronutrient Primer

When you consume food you are essentially putting raw materials into your body. Your body will then take these raw materials and use some of them for energy, some of them for building muscle and other tissues, and some of them to help create the hormones and other biochemistry needed to properly operate your body.

All food falls into one or more of the three main macronutrient types: Carbohydrates

Typically used for energy, carbohydrates are found in fruits, vegetables, nuts, and many processed foods. All carbohydrates break down into glucose in your bloodstream. Glucose is blood sugar and your body uses this to provide energy to your cells. In order to get the glucose out of your bloodstream and into your cells, your body must release insulin into your bloodstream as well. The unfortunate side efect of this is that the minute insulin spikes, fat storage begins.

Fats

Fats are essential to your health and have gotten a bad rap in the main-stream press. However, it has been proven that dietary fat does not make you produce body fat. Instead, fat helps your brain function, provides a secondary energy source, and perhaps most importantly it tells your body when you are full so that you don't overeat. These 'good' fats come from avocados, coconut oil, extra virgin olive oil, and some nuts. Additionally, the natural animal fats that come from beef, chicken, pork and some fsh are all perfectly fne and can be consumed on this diet.

+++++++++++++++++++++++++++++++

45

Protein

Proteins are the building blocks of muscle and are essential to your diet.

Without protein in your diet your muscles would waste away and you would eventually be unable to move.

Now that you understand the three macronutrients you are ready to learn how to combine them so that your body operates at its maximum efciency.

In this diet I always eat a protein choice, along with a vegetable selection, and a natural fat selection.

This is the macronutrient ratio that works very well in helping me maintain high energy levels, lose weight, and still feel satisfed and not hungry during the day:

Protein: 25% of daily calories

Carbs: 10% of daily calories

Fat: 65% of daily calories

I highly recommend that you fll up your daily meals with foods from the following seven main categories:

Meat and Eggs

Meat and eggs are of vital importance as they are the primary supplier of protein. Protein is essential since it is used to build and preserve the muscles on our body. Personally, while you may or may not want to build muscle, it's important that you preserve the muscle you do have. Muscle is metabolically active, meaning that the more you have, the faster your metabolism will be. In addition, muscle provides the underlying curves and lines that most people fnd attractive.

++++++++++++++++++++++++++++++++

46

Examples:

• Beef (grass fnished is best)

• Chicken (free range from local grower is best)

• Salmon (wild caught is best)

• Halibut (wild caught is best)

• Pork (if cured, make sure to fnd low sodium varieties) • Bacon (low sodium cured)

• Eggs (I suggest organic or farm grown eggs)

Vegetables

Vegetables are nature's suppliers of many vital nutrients…both vitamins and minerals. It is always best to select from the vegetable list, particularly the dark green, leafy variety, to get the most benefcial nutrients in your diet.

Examples:

- Spinach

- Chili Peppers

- Avocados

- Beets

- Broccoli

- Winter Squash

- Zucchini

- Kale

- Swiss Chard

- Brussels Sprouts

- Green Beans

- Asparagus

- Celery

- Carrots

++++++++++++++++++++++++++++++

47

Fruit

Fruits are a rich source of many antioxidants and other important vitamins and minerals. I recommend the following fruits be on the top of your weekly shopping list:

Examples:

- Tomatoes

- Bananas

- Cantaloupe

- Grapes

- Kiwi

- Oranges

- Nectarines

- Apples

Nuts

One of nature's most tasty sources of good fats, the nuts in this list will help you not only feel full, but they also provide great nutrient value as well.

Examples:

- Pistachios

- Almonds

- Brazil Nuts

++++++++++++++++++++++++++++++

48

Spices

Using herbs and spices is a healthy way to add favor to your plate, without adding sodium.

Examples:

- Dried Spearmint

- Dried Thyme

• Dried Dill

• Celery Seed

Oils

Whether used for cooking, marinades or salad dressing, healthy oils are always benefcial.

Examples:

• Coconut Oil

Drinks

Herbal teas contain an abundance of essential nutrients, and can be a refreshing drink, served hot or cold.

Examples:

• Hibiscus Tea

• Oolong Tea

• Hawthorn Berry Tea

+++++++++++++++++++++++++++++++

49

The complete food list is included in the Bonus Materials, "99 Foods that Naturally Lower Blood Pressure", which can be found in the back of this manual.

A word about the DASH diet

One diet you may have heard a lot about is the DASH diet. This diet was created by the National Institutes of Health and has won wide-ranging acclaim for its positive impact on lowering high blood pressure. If you would like more info on this diet I would encourage you to do a simple search for 'Dash diet", and you will fnd a plethora of resources.

I would caution you to be careful with the DASH diet however. It does recommend a lot of very good suggestions, however it still roughly follows the debunked Food Pyramid that was so boldly promoted by the U.S. government for years. The inclusion of whole grains, and the restriction of dietary fat is a deal killer for me. I have witnessed frst hand the negative impact of consuming too carbs from grain based products, which makes it impossible for me to honestly support that recommendation. In addition, I have also witnessed frst hand the very positive health benefts that one can achieve from increasing the amount of fat in your diet, while removing processed foods. I simply cannot ignore what I've seen and experienced frst hand, so therefore I can't wholeheartedly recommend the DASH diet.

++++++++++++++++++++++++++++++

50

Final Note

If you have more than 10lbs to lose you might want to checkout the PaleoBurn Fat Burner System. This comprehensive fat loss system is what I used to drop 31 lbs. of fat from my body, which contributed greatly to my success in getting my own high blood pressure under control. The full PaleoBurn program is designed to teach you how to quickly and safely lose fat from your body in a way that leaves you feeling full, with plenty of energy, and at the same time give you all the essential nutrients needed for optimal health.

Check it out here: paleoburn.com/bps

Resources:

1. n.a. "Most Americans Consume Too Much Sodium". Centers for Disease Control and Prevention.USA.gov. April 12, 2013. April 23, 2013.

http://www.cdc.gov/bloodpressure/sodium.htm

2. Suz. "The DASH Diet". The Paleo Network. May 1, 2012. April 23, 2013.

http://paleo.com.au/2012/05/dash-diet/

3. http://ajcn.nutrition.org/search?
author1=Loren+Cordain&sortspec=date&submit=Submit"Cordain, Loren Janette Brand Miller, S Boyd Eaton, Neil Mann, Susanne HA Holt, and John D Speth. "Plant-animal subsistence ratios and macronutrient energy estimations in worldwide hunter-gatherer diets". The American Journal of Clinical Nutrition. American Society for Clinical Nutrition. vol. 71 no. 3 682-692. March 2000. April 23, 2013.

http://ajcn.nutrition.org/content/71/3/682.long#fn-1

+++++++++++++++++++++++++++++++

51

Category 2: Smart Supplementation

While I recommend getting as much of the blood

pressure lowering vitamins and minerals from the

foods you eat each day, sometimes that simply

isn't possible. So, in this section I will outline exactly what vitamins and minerals that I recommend if

you are serious about lowering your blood

pressure. Each of these has been highly

researched, and I've even included links to the

studies that show why they work.

The Critical Role Of Vitamins, Minerals and Herbs

To Control Blood Pressure

In this chapter I want to introduce you to a family of vitamins, minerals, and herbs that studies suggest will improve blood pressure. You will want to include as many of the recommended foods as possible into your daily diet, because they naturally contain these vitamins and minerals. Refer to the 99 Foods That Naturally Lower Blood Pressure report to get even more information on which food types naturally contain these benefcial nutrients. While I suggest getting as many of these in your daily diet as possible, it is also highly benefcial to add supplements to your diet to makes sure that you are getting enough of the nutrients listed below.

Potassium

Based on overall studies, researchers have found that "a reduced intake of sodium and increased intake of potassium could make an important contri-

+++++++++++++++++++++++++++++++

52

bution to the prevention of hypertension, especially in populations with elevated blood pressure." Potassium appears to actually weaken the efects of excessive sodium intake.

Just like sodium, potassium is fundamental in maintaining adequate fuid and electrolyte balance. This essential macro mineral is signifcant to our brain, nerve, heart, muscles, performance and bone strength. The current recommended amount of potassium needed for healthy adults is 4,700 mg/

day, which can be easily achieved by eating a balanced diet containing potassium-rich fruits and vegetables. Unfortunately, research indicates that on average, most American adults do not consume enough potassium to reach this recommended amount, necessary for adequate nutrition.

Potassium supplements are available, however we recommend seeking your doctors recommendation prior to using any dietary replacement, particularly in this instance, if you have any type of kidney issues. It is important to note that unlike a dietary supplement, it's virtually impossible to exceed a safe level of natural potassium intake from fruit and vegetable sources.

Resources:

1. http://dx.doi.org/10.1161/ 01.HYP.0000202568.01167.B6

2. n.p., "Top 10 Vegetables Highest in Potassium", Healthaliciousness.com, n.d., Web.

Mar 3013

3. Lauren Kaufmann, "Eight Natural Ways To Lower Blood Pressure", June 22, 2012, Health Fair, Mar 2013, http://www.healthfair.com/eight-natural-ways-lower-bloodpressure/

4. Lauryn Muller, RDA Guidelines for Potassium, Livestrong.com, June 15, 2011 Livestrong.com, LIVESTRONG

Foundation, http://www.livestrong.com/article/471819-rda-guidelines-for-potassium/, March 2013

+++++++++++++++++++++++++++++++

53

Magnesium

In a study from the University of Hertfordshire, researchers found that "magnesium supplements may ofer small but clinically signifcant reductions in blood pressure." Combined studies further indicated that dietary supplementation of magnesium may have an efect in reducing blood pressure, particularly in higher dosages, according to the university's senior lecturer and registered nutritionist, Lindsy Kass.

While a diet low in magnesium may contribute to a rise in your blood pressure, doctors recommend making dietary modifcations to include healthy fruits and vegetables in preference to supplementing your diet with extra magnesium to help prevent high blood pressure. As always though, this depends on the individual. If you cannot get the proper amount of magnesium through dietary means, supplementation is necessary.

As with many recent studies, investigators have found that those who included minerals such as magnesium and potassium as part of their normal dietary intake can receive the natural benefts of a decreased risk of hypertension.

Resources:

1. MLA Citation: University of Hertfordshire. "Magnesium lowers blood pressure,

study suggests."ScienceDaily, 13

Mar. 2012. Web. 5 Mar. 2013

2. n.p., WebMD, Hypertension/High Blood Pressure Health Center, May 8, 2012, Web, March 6, 2013

+++++++++++++++++++++++++++++++

54

Calcium

Calcium, the most abundant mineral in the body, is known to provide strength to our bones and teeth, but it also plays a lesser-known part as an electrolyte, important to several signifcant biological processes.

While less than 1% of our bodies calcium reserve is needed to perform these functions, there has been much interest in its potential efect in lowering blood pressure.

Studies indicate that those who maintain a healthy balanced diet, which includes foods containing calcium, magnesium and potassium, tend to avoid health issues associated with hypertension. On the contrary, those who do not meet a sufcient intake of calcium in their diets tend to have higher blood pressure rates. So despite receiving mixed results, many researchers indicate that ongoing studies are warranted with regard to the positive efects that calcium may have in reducing blood pressure.

Resources:

1. n.p., University of Maryland Medical Center, University of Maryland School of Medicine,

http://www.umm.edu/patiented/articles/what_lifestyle_changes_needed_control_high_

htm, March 6, 2013

2. Cathy Wong, About.com Alternative Medicine, Updated September 24, 2012, Web,

March 6, 2013.

http://altmedicine.about.com/cs/herbsvitaminsek/a/Hypertension.htm 3. n.p.,Dietary Supplement Fact Sheet: Calcium, Natural Institutes of Health, http://ods.od.nih.gov/factsheets/Calcium-HealthProfessional/, March 6, 2013

4. http://dx.doi.org/10.1161/01.HYP.6.5.639

+++++++++++++++++++++++++++++++

55

Anthocyanins

Anthocyanins are a powerful part of the group of favonoids, notable for giving fruits and vegetables their colors, such as red, purple, and blue. Many scientifc studies have been performed to verify the positive efects that anthocyanins have in lowering blood pressure. Based on data collected, they concluded that this favonoid, along with favones, were the major contributors to the successful results, in comparison to other subclasses of favonoids.

In having the natural ability to increase nitric oxide, experts agree that habitual consumption of foods containing this impressive favonoid, is therefore efective in providing a reduction in blood pressure levels.

Scientists continue to strongly emphasize the importance of reducing blood pressure prior to reaching middle age. Considering the encouraging data provided in these studies, and having anthocyanin-rich foods readily available, consuming tea, grapes, blueberries, pomegranate, strawberries, eggplant and other similar food types, would be a safe and efective method for naturally reducing blood pressure levels.

Resources:

1. William Davis, MD, "Reduce Blood Pressure—Naturally-What Americans Can Learn from Traditional Cultures about Managing Hypertension", Life Extension Magazine,March 2010, Web, pg 1-2, March 2013

2. http://dx.doi.org/10.3945/"http://dx.doi.org/10.3945/ ajcn.110.006783

3. Jessica Bertrand, Flavonoids and Cardiovascular Health. AH-A, Agri-Food For Healthy Aging. Oct. 23, 2012.

March 2013. http://aha.the-ria.ca/blog/?p=1250

++++++++++++++++++++++++++++++++

56

Garlic

Garlic has been the subject of research studies for many years. Scientists have linked the use of garlic to having positive efects in regard to reducing cholesterol and blood pressure, among other benefts. Some have said that garlic is comparable in efectiveness to many antihypertensive medications such as beta-blocker, ACE inhibitors and ARBs (angiotensin II type 1 receptor antagonists). Garlic has shown to have the ability to relax blood vessels and thin the blood, however there are concerns regarding the risk of potential drug interactions, such as Coumadin, which also have blood-thinning properties.

There has been much debate among experts regarding the specifc form of garlic, with respect to it's safety and efectiveness in treating such conditions as high cholesterol and blood pressure. However, despite conficting opinions, most studies have concluded that garlic has shown to be benefcial to some degree, having a positive efect in lowering blood pressure whether ingested through foods or natural supplements.

Some experts believe that consuming raw garlic is most efective, due to diminishing benefts once cooked. Others indicate that while positive health benefts can be achieved, consuming large amounts of raw garlic for medicinal purposes may cause tolerable gastrointestinal side efects, not to mention the unpleasant odor, which many fnd unpleasant.

Over the years, many studies have indicated that allicin, a component of garlic, responsible for it's distinctive aromatic properties, may be the key to the herb's efectiveness in treating hypertension. However, there have recently been difering opinions regarding whether or not allicin should be
++++++++++++++++++++++++++++++++

considered to be the contributor to garlic's success. Citing the chemical instability of the enzyme once ingested, many professionals now believe that aged garlic extract (AGE), which contains the active and stable component S-allylcysteine, allows for a standardized dosage, and shows to be the most efective form of garlic when considering it for use in lowering blood pressure.

A recent study was published in the European Journal of Clinical Nutrition, in which researchers assessed the efectiveness of aged garlic extract for use by those currently experiencing uncontrolled blood pressure, in conjunction with their prescribed medications for hypertension.

There were 79 participants included in the study, each having uncontrolled systolic hypertension. They were given a quantity of aged garlic extract based on a daily dosage of one capsule (240 mg containing 0.6 mg of S-allylcysteine), two capsules (480 mg with 1.2 mg of S-allylcysteine), four capsules (960 mg containing 2.4 mg of S-allylcysteine), or a placebo.

Results indicated that those in the 2-capsule group experienced a signifcant reduction in systolic blood pressure over 12 weeks compared with the placebo, while the 4-capsule group reached borderline reduction at 8

weeks. There was no signifcant diference however in the 1-capsule group and diastolic pressure. Researchers concluded that the aged garlic extract should be considered as a safe and efective treatment for those with uncontrolled hypertension, in conjunction with antihypertensive therapies, as prescribed.

+++++++++++++++++++++++++++++++

Overall, studies confrm that garlic has shown to be benefcial in lowering blood pressure, with most recent results indicating the success of using aged garlic extract as a safe and efective treatment.

Resources:

1. Christopher Hobbs, LAc, AHG. "The Heart Herbs: Hawthorn and Garlic". Healthy.net. n.d. Mar. 18, 2013.

http://www.healthy.neHYPERLINK "http://www.healthy.net/scr/article.aspx?Id=899"t http://www.healthy.net/scr/article.aspx?Id=899"/scr/article.aspx?Id=899

2. Dr. Simi Paknikar, "Garlic Lowers Blood Pressure in Hypertensive Patients". MedIndia. Health In Focus. Jan. 10, 2012. Mar. 19, 2013 http://www.medindia.net/news/healthinfocus/Garlic-Lowers-BloodPressure-in-Hypertensive-Patients-95906-1.htm

3. Carmia Borek, PhD. Aged Garlic Extract Lowers Blood Pressure.Total Health Magazine.com.The Wellness Imperative.n.d. March 19, 2013.

http://totalhealthmagazine.com/articles/cardiovascular-health/aged-garlic-extract-lowers-bloodpressure.html 4. http://dx.doi.org/10.1038/ejcn.2012.178

Selenium

Selenium, a trace mineral, is an essential micronutrient. As a component of an unusual group of amino acids, selenium works as an antioxidant, important to protecting our bodies on a cellular level.

Evidence suggests that selenium, shown to be efective in preventing infam-matory diseases, may also be efective in protecting against other conditions, such as atherosclerosis (vascular disease) and hypertension.

+++++++++++++++++++++++++++++

59

Much research has been done on the efectiveness of selenium supplementation as a prevention of many diseases, but indicates rather that for most Americans, this is not necessary, as sufcient amounts of the mineral are found in dietary sources.

After conducting a study, Dr. Larry C. Clark at the University of Arizona warned that, "While the promise of beneft from a daily supplement is strong, it has not been proved, and the possibility of toxicity for those who overdo it is serious indeed."

Mustard products are an excellent source of selenium, as well as many other valuable nutrients including calcium, potassium, omega 3 fatty acids, and magnesium, just to name a few. Though the richest source of selenium can be found in Brazil nuts, with 1 ounce containing 537 mcg of selenium, which is 767% of daily nutritional value.

Resources:

1. Dietary Supplement Fact Sheet: Selenium, Ofce of Dietary Supplements, National Institutes of Health, October 12, 2012, March 13, 2013, http://ods.od.nih.gov/factsheets/Selenium-HealthProfessional/

http://ods.od.nih.gov/factsheets/Selenium-HealthProfessional/#h6/

2. Christine Roberts, "Pass the mustard and those health benefts please", NaturalNews.com, Wednesday, January 05, 2011, March 1, 2013, http://www.naturalnews.com/030916_mustard_health_food.html 3. Carla, "HEALTH BENEFITS OF MUSTARD SEEDS", Guide to Herbal Remedies, HERBAL REMEDIES AND NATURAL

HEALTH, January 15, 2010, Mar 1, 2013,

http://guide2herbalremedies.com/health-benefts-mustard-seeds/

4. The World's Healthiest Foods, The George Mateljan Foundation, n.d., ++++++++++++++++++++++++++++++

60

http://www.whfoods.com/genpage.php?tname=foodspice&dbid=106"

http://www.whfoods.com/genpage.php?tname=foodspice

http://www.whfoods.com/genpage.php?tname=foodspice&dbid=106"&

http://www.whfoods.com/genpage.php?tname=foodspice&dbid=106"dbid=106, Mar 2013

5. Jane E. Brody, "Hopes Rising for Selenium", Health-NY Times, Feb. 19, 1997, Web. Mar. 18, 2013.

http://www.nytimes.com/1997/02/19/us/hopes-rising-for-selenium.html?pagewanted=all http://www.nytimes.com/1997/02/19/us/hopes-rising-for-selenium.html?pagewanted=all&src=pm"&H

http://www.nytimes.com/1997/02/19/us/hopes-rising-for-selenium.html?
pagewanted=all&src=pm"src=pm

Nitrates

Nitrates, from dietary sources such as beets and leafy green vegetables, are converted to nitric oxide within our system. In response, the nitric oxide relaxes and dilates blood vessels. Research demonstrates that consuming foods rich in nitrates is efective in lowering blood pressure through a natural process of improving blood fow. Several studies have shown that beetroot juice, when consumed daily, can signifcantly reduce blood pressure levels in only 24 hrs. Scientists believe that this is a result of the nitrates, which naturally occur in foods such as beetroot juice.

Another study indicated that similar results were achieved in those given a nitrate supplement, though the study concluded that while the nitrate supplement did not reduce systolic blood pressure, it did have an efect in lowering diastolic blood pressure readings. In conclusion, scientists indicated that additional research was warranted.

Nitrates should not to be confused with nitrites, which are substances often used in curing meat.

+++++++++++++++++++++++++++++++++

Resources:

1. http://dx.doi.org/10.1016/j.niox.2009.10.007

2. Sophie Borland, Drinking beetroot juice dramatically lowers risk of heart disease and strokes, Published by Associated Newspapers Ltd Part of the Daily Mail, The Mail on Sunday & Metro Media Group, June 29, 2010, March 12, 2013, http://www.dailymail.co.uk/health/article-1290434/Drinking-beetroot-juice-dramatically-lowers-risk-heartdisease-strokes.html

3. Maye Hadson, Can Nitrates Help Control High Blood Pressure?, Zimbio, Lovingly

Media, Inc., July 22, 2011, March 12, 2013,
http://www.zimbio.com/High+Blood+Pressure/articles/Dtt0RD71ehu/Can+Nitrates+H
+High+Blood+Pressure

L-Arginine

L-Arginine is an amino acid naturally produced by the human body. Included in a team of other compounds, this amino acid participates in an important chemical reaction that produces nitric oxide. The inner lining of our blood vessels, (called the endothelium) uses the nitric oxide as a vasodilator (widening the walls of blood vessels, increasing blood fow), which is critical to key controlling high blood pressure.

Scientists have shown that vascular disease can be identifed as a result of endothelial dysfunction, which causes hypertension, and is associated with numerous other diseases such as heart disease and diabetes, as well. So researchers conclude that the presence of L-Arginine, as it relates to the production of nitric oxide, is a good indicator of healthy endothelial cells, thereby helping to decrease high blood pressure in clinical hypertensive patients.

++++++++++++++++++++++++++++++++

62

Researchers suggest that while our bodies naturally produce this amino acid, individuals with poor diets or particular health issues would benet by consuming foods containing arginine, including nuts, seeds, beef, pork, and poultry.

Resources:

1. http://dx.doi.org/10.1016/S0008-6363(99)00115-7

2. http://dx/doi.org/10.1097/00004872-200501000-00004

3. Gokce, N.. (October 2004). "L-Arginine and hypertension". Journal of Nutrition 134 (10 Suppl): 2807S–2811S

REVIEW. PMID http://www.ncbi.nlm.nih.gov/pubmed/15465790" 15465790

4. http://dx.doi.org/10.1161/ HYPERTENSIONAHA.108.114298

5. http://dx.doi.org/10.1016/j.ahj.2011.09.012

Sodium

The discussion on sodium must begin with the acceptance of four important facts:

1. Sodium is required for proper cell function inside your body. You simply cannot live without proper levels of sodium in your body.

2. Too much sodium is a major risk factor for high blood pressure 3. Table salt is the worst form of sodium you can put into your body.

4. There are other, more healthy alternatives to table salt that can allow you to still have the taste of salt.

+++++++++++++++++++++++++++++++

63

The truth is that your body requires

sodium to function properly.

Sodium is critical to maintaining

our body's health on a cellular level.

This essential mineral is needed to

neutralize the acids in our bodies

that can result from a poor diet and

a stressful lifestyle.

There is no doubt that too much

sodium of any kind is a contributing factor to high blood pressure. In fact, the ofcial stance on salt (table salt) from the American Heart Association recommends limiting sodium intake to no more than 1,500 milligrams a day. This is especially important for those with high risk factors such as those at the age of 51 or older, who are black, or who have existing high blood pressure, diabetes, or chronic kidney disease.

TIPS FOR LOWERING YOUR SODIUM INTAKE without sacrifcing favor in your foods:

• Replace the salt in your saltshaker with a few of your favorite seasonings, and if you're eating out, have some handy in a plastic bag or small container.

• There are also products that contain a

mixture of seasonings,

specifcally blended for

various types of meals,

which adds conve—

nience. But be careful

to read the label on all

seasonings, as many

also contain salt, which

you are trying to avoid.

+++++++++++++++++++++++++++++++

64

For those concerned with reducing their sodium intake, it's important to consider that the primary source of our "bad" sodium intake can be found in most every type of pre-packaged and processed foods available, compared to that added to our dinner plate. Chemically processed foods are flled with "bad salt" that actually drains the electrolytes that our bodies need, thereby increasing the negative efects of a high sodium diet.Key to understanding the importance of our bodies need for sodium, is also knowing that just like fat, there are both good and bad types of this salty mineral.

Table salt is highly processed and has been stripped of the trace minerals that occur naturally in the healthy forms of salt such as the natural, unprocessed sea salts. No longer able to be properly absorbed by the body, in excess, these refned types of salt, along with the harmful additives they contain, can contribute to many health issues, including high blood pressure.

So is sodium good or bad for blood pressure?

Let's take a closer look.

Many believe that this recommendation comes as a warning to "put down the salt shaker", without understanding the biological necessity for including sodium as a part of a healthy diet.

However, It is in the over consumption of sodium that you get into trouble.

So, what is the best way to lower your consumption of sodium when the 'bad' type of sodium (the overly processed kind) is in so many foods that we eat. Also, what do you do when you want to still enjoy the taste of salt?

++++++++++++++++++++++++++++++

65

Natural Sea Salt To The Rescue:

Consider using natural sea salt. Unlike table salt, which is mined from the ground and typically referred to as mineral salt, natural sea salt is produced from the evaporation of seawater. Production of sea salt has been dated to prehistoric times. Consider that this "good salt" when used in moderation, is an acceptable choice for use in cooking and seasoning your healthy foods.

It's also important to know what to look for when searching for the healthy alternative, which is raw, unrefned sea salt. You might fnd a wide variety of sea salt options, so it's best to always check the label. If it's white in color, or is made entirely of sodium chloride, then it's been refned/processed. What you're looking for should be one that has color (pink, grey, etc.), and lists plenty of trace minerals.

While it is true that most brands of sea salt contain roughly the same amount of sodium as table salt, it also contains many of the trace elements such as potassium that balance the levels of sodium in your system.

In addition, there are certain brands of sea salts that are processed in a special way to reduce the amount of sodium intake by as much as 57%.

Visit BloodPressureSolution.com/seasalt for more info on this highly recommended sea salt.

Onion, garlic, cumin, and chili powders, as well as cracked black pepper are some of the most commonly used spices, but there are plenty of options when looking for ways to replace the sodium with a healthy dose of favor.

Here are a few antioxidant rich seasonings you might like to try: • Cayenne pepper; great for any food if you like to spice things up • Oregano or marjoram; (add to salads, soups, tomato-based sauces) • Dried mint; (great for salad, tea, and also adds a sweet favor to water) • Parsley; (great for most savory dishes, salads, and even blended into a protein shake)

• Cinnamon or cloves (great to add a little spice to a sweet potato)

Resources:

1. Katherine Zeratsky, R.D., L.D., Nutrition and healthy eating, "What's the diference between sea salt and table salt?", MayoClinic.com, Mayo Foundation for Medical Education and Research, http://www.mayoclinic.com/health/seasalt/AN01142, Mar 5, 2013

2. Shannon, Simplebites.net, Simple Living Media, Feb 25, 2010, Web, Mar 6, 2013

3. ANN LOUISE GITTLEMAN, N.D., M.S., Understanding Salt and Sodium,, n.p. , n.d., Web, March 5, 2013

Capsaicin

Capsaicin, included as part of the capsaicinoids family, is responsible for the heat found in foods such as cayenne and red peppers, has been shown to be efective in reducing blood pressure, and overall heart health.

Zhen-Yu Chen, Ph.D., who presented the study, indicated, "We now have a clearer and more detailed portrait of their innermost efects on genes and other mechanisms that infuence cholesterol and the health of blood vessels. It is among the frst research to provide that information."

Other studies confrm fnding, showing that both systolic and diastolic blood pressures were reduced after long term consumption of dietary capsaicin.

By detecting the human protein that regulates body temperature, capsaicin is efective in increasing energy and reducing fat storage in those who included foods containing this fery hot substance as part of a healthy diet.

In addition to capsaicin, cayenne peppers are also high in vitamins A, B

complex, and C. Cayenne peppers are also rich in both calcium and potassium, both of which are minerals shown to have an efect on lowering blood pressure.

Resources:

1. MLA: American Chemical Society (ACS). "Hot pepper compound could help hearts."ScienceDaily, 27 Mar. 2012.

Web. 28 Feb. 2013.

2. http://dx.doi.org/10.1016/j.cmet.2010.05.015

3. http://dx.doi.org/10.1038/39807

4. http://dx.doi.org/10.1016/j.cub.2011.01.031

Coenzyme Q10

Coenzyme Q10 (abbreviated as CoQ10) is a vitamin-like substance needed for proper cell function. Our bodies naturally produce CoQ10, which is highly concentrated in several of our major organs, particularly the heart.

Author and nutrition expert Keri Glassman, confrms that researchers are excited to discover the importance of ubiquinol (the converted form of CoQ10), relative to maintaining cardiovascular health. According to Glassman, "CoQ10 and ubiquinol levels diminish with age…making cells more vulnerable to cell damage."

Scientists have found that CoQ10 has a positive efect in reducing cardiovascular complications, also indicating that those with previous heart-related conditions were defcient in this powerful enzyme.

There has also been much interest in CoQ10 and how it afects blood pressure. Several studies indicate that those given CoQ10 supplements twice daily signifcantly reduced both systolic and diastolic blood pressures.

Some believe that adding a CoQ10 supplementation, in addition to efective diet and lifestyle changes, can reduce the need for prescribing multiple medications for those experiencing high blood pressure. Since CoQ10 is produced naturally in the human body, there are virtually no side efects resulting from supplementation of this antioxidant.

Resources:

1. William Davis, MD, "Reduce Blood Pressure—Naturally-What Americans Can Learn from Traditional Cultures about Managing Hypertension", Life Extension Magazine, March 2010, Web, pg 1-2, March 2013

2. Cathy Wong, About.com Alternative Medicine, Updated September 24, 2012, Web, March 12, 2013

3. http://dx.doi.org/10.3949/ccjm.77a.09078"doi.org/10.3949/ccjm.77a.09078

4. Keri Glassman, "5 Things You Can Do This Month To Make Your Heart Healthier". Nutritious Life.com. Feb. 14, 2013. Mar. 18, 2013.

http://www.nutritiouslife.com/nlts/5-things-you-can-do-this-month-to-make-your-heart-healthier/

++++++++++++++++++++++++++++++

69

Omega-3

Omega-3 is a fatty acid, which is not naturally produced by our bodies. The two types of Omega-3 are EPA and DHA. This fatty acid can be commonly found in fsh, as well as other food sources such as fresh fruits and vegetables, olive oil, garlic, various types of both seeds and nuts.

Fish oils have been the topic of much research regarding its efect in reducing high blood pressure by expanding the blood vessels. Studies have also been conducted which indicate that the intake of Omega-3 also promotes cardiovascular health, improving weight loss and decreasing blood sugar, in addition to other diseases.

Many researchers suggest that for those with existing hypertension, maintaining a low fat diet while consuming foods rich in Omega-3 fatty acid, or with supplementation, would warrant consideration as an efective way to reduce blood pressure.

According to Dr. Jeremiah Stamler, professor emeritus of preventive medicine at Northwestern University in Chicago, "A large percentage of people between ages 20 and 60 have a rise in blood pressure, and by middle age many have high blood pressure." Based on the results of his study, he indicated that further research would be done in order to focus on the "dietary factors that may help prevent that rise, and omega-3 fatty acids are a small, but important piece of the action," he said.

The study review results confrmed that there were signifcant reductions in both the systolic and diastolic blood pressure. While there were insignifcant
++++++++++++++++++++++++++++++

70

results for those who did not have high blood pressure, the positive results achieved from the hypertensive group were encouraging.

This review confrmed previous conclusions of the positive efects of using Omega-3, as a supplement or via natural food sources, for those with hypertension, and potentially with those with other cardiovascular diseases.

However, for those who are currently taking prescribed antihypertensive medications, it is important to consult a physician prior to including any Omega-3 supplementation, as this could result in a dangerous reduction in blood pressure levels.

Resources:

1. J.D. Heyes. Lower Your Blood Pressure Signifcantly with Omega-3 Fatty Acids. Natural News Network. Truth Publishing International, LTD. Sunday, Dec. 30, 2012. March 27, 2013.

http://www.naturalnews.com/038507_blood_pressure_omega-3_fatty_acids.html 2. http://dx.doi.org/10.1161, http://dx.doi.org/10.1161/ 01.HYP.22.3.371

3. http://dx.doi.org/10.1177/2047487312437056

Hawthorne

Hawthorn, rich in favonoids, is an herb, which has been used successfully for centuries to treat cardiovascular conditions by efectively aiding in blood circulation. No herb-drug interactions were reported.

Christopher Hobbs, a fourth generation herbalist and botanist with over 30

years experience with herbs refers to hawthorn as "The best-known herb for
++++++++++++++++++++++++++++++++

71

the heart in western herbalism…available in capsules or tablets in the U.S.

and other parts of the world."

Quercetin and oligomeric procyanidins (OPCs), the same antioxidants found in grapes, are among the types of favonoids that may be responsible for hawthorn's efectiveness, according to a study by University of Maryland University Medical Center.

According to Dr. James Meschino, recognized as a leading expert in nutrition, anti-aging, ftness and wellness, "Scientifc and clinical investigations have shown that active constituents in hawthorn extract can reduce high blood pressure via their infuence on the angiotensin system, by acting as calcium channel blockers and by improving endothelial function. When taken with coenzyme Q10, and in conjunction with other antihypertensive lifestyle measures, hawthorn supplementation is a key element in the natural management of mild to moderate high blood pressure."

In an online forum found in Men's Health regarding blood pressure issues, a hypertensive male reported to have received excellent results in reducing his blood pressure levels after 5 weeks of using hawthorn, which he had purchased at a local chain retailer. He indicated that within a weeks time of not using the hawthorn, his blood pressure began to noticeably increase. He stated that upon reintroducing the hawthorn supplement, his blood pressure began to decrease again after only a few days, confrming the efectiveness of this herbal supplement from his personal experience.

++++++++++++++++++++++++++++++++

Resources:

1. Dr. James Meschino, DC, MS, ND, ROHP, RAP. "Hawthorn, The Three-In-One Natural Remedy For High Blood Pressure. Meschino Health.com. n.d. Mar. 18, 2013.

http://www.meschinohealth.com/ArticleDirectory/Hawthorn_Natural_Blood_Pressure 2. Dr. CathyWong, "Natural Remedies for High Blood Pressure". About.com Guide, Sept. 24, 2012. Mar. 18, 2013:
http://altmedicine.about.com/cs/herbsvitaminsek/a/Hypertension.htm 3. Christopher Hobbs, LAc, AHG. "The Heart Herbs: Hawthorn and Garlic". Healthy.net. n.d. Mar. 18, 2013.

http://www.healthy.net/scr/article.aspx?Id=899

4. Blood Pressure Issues (Sept. 7, 2006). [online forum comment]. Retrieved from http://forums.menshealth.com/eve/forums/a/tpc/f/789103123/m/3241015711

Olive Leaf Extract

The medicinal benefts of the leaves of the olive tree have been known since ancient times. Research studies are now fnding that a supplement containing the ingredients found in olive leaf extract, may be an efective therapy for many health conditions, including for those hypertension.

A study was conducted including 20 sets of identical twins, each considered to be "borderline" hypertensive. Give 1,000 mg of olive leaf extract per day resulted in a signifcant reduction in both their overall blood pressure readings, as well as LDL ("bad" cholesterol) levels, in only 8 weeks. The study participants who did not receive the supplements did not show a signifcant change in blood pressure.

++++++++++++++++++++++++++++++++

73

Researchers believe that the relaxing efect to the walls of the arteries may have been a result of a combination of ingredients found in the olive leaf extract. Olive leaves contain secoiridoids, which include ligustroside, oleacein, and most importantly oleuropein. The high concentrations of oleuropein are what researchers believe are the most signifcant compound in reducing blood pressure readings. The properties of oleuropein show to have a direct efect on the stifness and resistance of arteries, aiding in improving the function of the inner lining of blood vessels, and regulating blood pressure.

Based on the positive evidence from the study, health professionals recommend taking 500 mg of olive leaf extract, twice daily. Please do not stop taking any prescribed medications, or take olive leaf supplements, without prior consultation with your physician.

Apple Cider Vinegar

Apple Cider vinegar, made from apple cider, is available in both a raw and processed form. Many health experts recommend using the organic, unprocessed apple cider vinegar, which is referred to as "mother" on the label.

This unfltered form contains strands that many believe are responsible for its benefcial qualities as a natural treatment for a wide variety of conditions.

In addition to being efective at treating the symptoms of common colds, infections, and skin problems, this miracle liquid is said to have positive ef-fects for weight control, and improving both cholesterol and blood pressure readings.

++++++++++++++++++++++++++++++++

74

Apple cider vinegar contains an array of various vitamins and minerals, including potassium, sodium, magnesium, calcium, and phosphorous. It is believed that the successful results of using this vinegar as a natural treatment for lowering blood pressure is due to these vital nutrients.

There are many testimonials touting the amazing results achieved, including one indicating a drop of 20 points in systolic blood pressure and 30 points in diastolic, over period of about of three months.

The average recommended dosage is one glass of water daily, with ~2 tablespoons of raw, organic apple cider vinegar. It's important to note that due to the highly acidic nature of apple cider vinegar, it should always be diluted to avoid the potential of eroding tooth enamel, or burning your throat. Most who regularly use this treatment were honest in stating that the taste can be somewhat unpleasant, but the benefts far outweigh the ofensive taste and smell.

To improve this problem, some suggested adding the apple cider vinegar to a small glass of juice initially, though this can greatly increase the sugar/carb content. Another recommendation was to add stevia, a natural sweetener, with 2 tablespoons of the vinegar to a glass of water, which also improved the taste.

While there have been no reported harmful efects of using apple cider vinegar, it is always best to consult your physician prior to making changes to your dietary health plan.

++++++++++++++++++++++++++++++++

75

Resources:

1. Mullins, Brittany (2012, Feb. 20). "Health Benefts of Apple Cider Vinegar (ACV)". [weblog post] Retrieved from http://www.eatingbirdfood.com/2012/02/health-benefts-of-apple-cider-vinegar-acv/

2. Kevin Mathias. "Health Benefts of Apple Cider Vinegar". Buzzle.com. Updated 1/2/2013. April 20, 2013.

http://www.buzzle.com/articles/health-benefts-apple-cider-vinegar.html 3. Wendler, Jim. (2012, Dec. 19).Blood Pressure Remedy-Apple Cider Vinegar.[weblog post] Retrieved from http://www.jimwendler.com/2011/12/bloodpressure-remedy-apple-cider-vinegar/

4. Lori L. "Apple Cider Vinegar for High Blood Pressure Treatment-Part 2 in a series about Apple Cider Vinegar…"

Natural Healing Remedies. November 15, 2009. April 20, 2013.

http://naturalhealingremedies.org/index.php/2009/11/apple-cider-vinegar-for-highblood-pressure-treatment/

Vitamin C

Vitamin C, commonly touted as being efective in fghting the common cold, is benefcial for so many other reasons… one of which is associated with hypertension. Studies have shown that for those with mild to moderate hypertension, this antioxidant vitamin is benefcial in reducing blood pressure readings.

Researchers cited that the notable efects were seen in those taking a dosage higher than that which is considered to be a recommended daily requirement. For those taking ~500 milligrams of vitamin C, their blood pressure readings dropped by nearly 5 millimeters.

++++++++++++++++++++++++++++++++

76

From these fndings, researchers confrmed that the blood vessel walls were relaxed, which resulted in the blood pressure reduction, due to the natural diuretic efects of vitamin C, involving the process of removing sodium and water from the body.

Studies also concluded that vitamin C was efective in restoring the elasticity in blood vessel walls, aiding in the prevention of plaque formation.

When looking for a vitamin C supplement, health experts suggest the added benefts of choosing one that is in combination with other vitamins and minerals, such as vitamin E, calcium, magnesium, and iron.

While the daily-recommended dosage of vitamin C is 60 milligrams, an increased dosage is suggested, due to a general lack of vitamin C consumed in the average diet. Supplementation of up to 500 milligrams per day may prove to have the most blood pressure lowering efects, though a dosage of 200-300 milligrams per day would promote a general sense of better health.

Resources:

1. Dr. Andrew Weil, M.D. High Blood Pressure, Hypertension. Condition Care Guide. Weil Lifestyle. Updated 8/30/2012. April 19, 2013. http://www.drweil.com/drw/u/ART00686/highblood-pressure-treatment 2. John Phillip.Vitamin C lowers blood pressure, improves vascular function to lower heart attack and stroke risk".

NaturalNews.com. Natural News Network. Sept. 12, 2012. April 19, 2013.

http://www.naturalnews.com/037163_vitamin_c_blood_pressure_heart_attack_risk.htr 3. http://dx.doi.org/10.3945/ ajcn.111.027995

++++++++++++++++++++++++++++++

77

Vitamin E

Vitamin E, a fat-soluble nutrient, is benefcial to protecting your body on a cellular level. This antioxidant can be found in many foods, including vegetables such as spinach and broccoli, in fruits such as kiwi and mangos, as well as many seeds and nuts.

Like other antioxidant vitamins such as vitamins A and C, vitamin E may play an important role in protecting your body from the cell damage caused by environmental free radicals such as cigarette smoke, and air pollution.

Vitamin E also has properties benefcial to hypertension, in that is involved in the process of creating red blood cells, helps to widen and prevent blood clotting in the vessels.

There have been some conficting results in response to claims that vitamin E has the ability to prevent cancer, heart disease, and other related health issues, but many studies did confrm that further studies were warranted.

However, one study did conclude encouraging results for women. Researchers found that among study participants taking vitamin E, the women had a 24% reduction in cardiovascular death rates. Additionally, in a group of those 65 years of age and older, results showed a decrease in non-fatal heart attacks, and a signifcant decrease in cardiovascular deaths, as well.

Vitamin E defciency is rare in most individuals, so health experts agree that getting adequate amounts of vitamin E from natural food sources is best.

But supplementation is another option, if you do not get adequate dietary amounts, or if you have certain health conditions and are not able to properly digest the fat required to properly absorb the nutrient.

+++++++++++++++++++++++++++++++

78

It's important to note that vitamin

E is often mistakenly referred

to as being a single substance,

though there are actually several

naturally occurring forms of the

vitamin. So when choosing a

vitamin E supplement, it is

suggested that you look for those listed as "d-alpha-tocopherol", which comes from a natural source. Others included in the group of natural forms of vitamin E are d-beta-, and d-gamma-tocopherol, or may be labeled as "mixed tocopherols". Some multi-vitamins, which contain vitamin E and other essential nutrients, are also available. Be sure to check the label, and avoid any supplement containing synthetic forms of nutrients, with the vitamin E listed as "dl-" forms, which are less potent.

Vitamin E supplementation IS NOT RECOMMENDED if:

• ...You are considering taking high amounts of vitamin E-this can be harmful. The highest safe level for adults of

vitamin E in natural form

is 1,500 IUs a day and

1,000 IUs/day for synthetic supplement form.

• …You have been diagnosed with any condition

such as Crohn's disease,

cystic fbrosis, or certain

genetic diseases

• …You are undergoing

chemotherapy or radia—

tion therapy

• …You are taking any

blood thinning medication, such as Coumadin,

as vitamin E can increase

your risk for bleeding.

+++++++++++++++++++++++++++++++

79

Currently, the recommended daily allowance for natural vitamin E (d-alpha-tocopherol, d-beta-tocopherol) for males age 14+ years is 15 mg (22.4 IU), and for females age 14+ years is 15 mg (22.4 IU).

Health professionals do warn against certain health risks involved with taking vitamin E supplements with regard to possible drug interactions and health conditions. As always, it is important to talk to your doctor to decide what option is best for you prior to taking any

Dietary supplement.

Resources:

1. Boshtam M, Rafei M, Sadeghi K, Sarraf-Zadegan N."Vitamin E can reduce blood pressure in mild hypertensives". National Center for Biotechnology Information, U.S. National Library of Medicine.October 2002.

April 20, 2013. http://www.ncbi.nlm.nih.gov/pubmed/12463106

2. n.a. "Dietary Supplement Fact Sheet: Vitamin E". NIH Ofce of Dietary Supplements.

Reviewed October 11, 2011. April 20, 2013. http://ods.od.nih.gov/factsheets/VitaminE-QuickFacts/?print=1

3. n.a. "Dietary Supplement Fact Sheet: Vitamin E:. NIH Ofce of Dietary Supplements.

Reviewed October 11, 2011. April 20, 2013. http://ods.od.nih.gov/factsheets/VitaminE-HealthProfessional/

4. Lee I-M, Cook NR, Gaziano JM, Gordon D, Ridker PM, Manson JE, "Vitamin E in the primary prevention of cardiovascular disease and cancer: the Women's Health Study: a randomized controlled trial" July 6, 2005.

April 20, 2013. http://www.ncbi.nlm.nih.gov/pubmed/15998891?dopt=Abstract 5. n.a. "Facts about Vitamin E". Healing Edgs Sciences, Inc. n.d. April 20, 2013.

http://www.healingedge.net/store/article_vitamin_e.html

6. Dr. Joseph Mercola. "Eliminate This Everyday Food and Watch Your High Blood Pressure Plunge".

October 8, 2010. April 20, 2013.

http://articles.mercola.com/sites/articles/archive/2010/10/08/discover-the-secret-to-lowering-your-bloodpressure-in-15-minutes.aspx

---

++++++++++++++++++++++++++++++++

80

Vitamin D3

Vitamin D is well known for its wonders of working with calcium in building strong bones, and keeping them healthy as you age. Now scientists are showing that Vitamin D is signifcant to the process of many other important biological functions. Of great importance is its role in the process of angio-genesis (which involves your body's ability to grow new blood vessels from your pre-existing ones).

But without adequate amounts of vitamin D, your biological stores begin to decrease. This defciency triggers your body to release increasing amounts of specifc hormones, and as a result your blood pressure is elevated.

Scientifc studies have concluded that vitamin D defciency has been associated with a group of health problems, including insulin resistance, obesity, and hypertension. In addition to it's involvement in regulating your immune system, (relevant due to its ability to decrease infammation), vitamin D has also been shown to reduce systolic blood pressure, and is a requirement for statins (drugs prescribed to lower cholesterol levels) to work efectively, as well.

There are several factors that can determine the adequacy of your vitamin D intake, the most signifcant of which is your exposure to sunlight. But variables such as your personal climate, as well as the season, and the amount of time you spend outdoors, and even your skin color should be considered.

And with the responsible use of sunscreen, (important for reducing your risk of skin cancer due to sun exposure), this too can afect the benefts you receive from that exposure.

++++++++++++++++++++++++++++++++

81

According to one published study, the authors indicated that blacks appeared to have signifcantly higher rates of hypertension than whites, as well as lower levels of vitamin D present.

The results of the study showed that after 3 months of vitamin D3 supplementation, lower blood pressure readings were achieved. Researchers agreed that further trials were warranted with regard to vitamin D supplementation and its blood pressure lowering efects in the black population, in order to determine a direct link between the two factors. The diferences in numbers were modest, yet signifcant, which were said to be promising news.

Research has shown that an estimated 50-70% of Europeans may be defcient in vitamin D. A group of Danish researchers conducted a small study, and found that the participants taking the vitamin D supplement showed a signifcant reduction in central systolic blood pressure readings.

Additional results showed that for those originally defcient in vitamin D, there was a slight reduction in ambulatory blood pressure, which was of borderline signifcance. The scientists concluded that as a result of this study hypertensive patients, who are defcient in vitamin D, could beneft from supplementation. They further stated that while not to be considered a cure for high blood pressure, it may prove to be especially helpful during the winter months (or times when adequate sun exposure is not available).

In addition to good old-fashioned sunlight, another primary source of vitamin D is from natural foods, both of which cause your body to produce naturally. Foods that contain highest levels of vitamin D include wild salmon,
++++++++++++++++++++++++++++++++

82

tuna, sardines, Pacifc founder, sole or white cod fsh, pork, eggs, Shiitake mushrooms, beef, almond milk (the same amount as dairy milk), green leafy vegetables, broccoli, papaya, and orange juice.

If you are not able to get sufcient amounts of vitamin D through natural sources of sunlight or foods, then supplements are another option. However, it is important to choose D3 (cholecalciferol) supplements, which are more efective than the synthetic form D2 (ergocalciferol). Also, most prescribed forms of vitamin D contain D2 (synthetic), so request D3 for the most beneft.

It is also very important to note that taking too much vitamin D can cause a dangerous overdose. For this reason sunlight and food sources are the best choice, in that it's practically impossible to receive too much of vitamin D

from these natural sources.

Before choosing whether or not to take a D3 supplement, it is very important that you visit your doctor, in order to get an accurate reading of your body's current level of vitamin D. This can only be determined by a blood test, through your doctor. Due to the environmental factors, the color of your skin, the amount of vitamin D you receive from sun exposure and your diet, safely determining accurate dosage requirements should be based on your test results.

The U.S. RDA for vitamin D is 400 IU, is based on the amount necessary to prevent diseases such as rickets, which is sufcient. However, in order to achieve the beneft of protection for heart disease and other associated conditions, a much a higher dosage is required.

++++++++++++++++++++++++++++++++

83

But according to the most recent studies, 35 IU's of vitamin D, per pound of body weight, is the currently recommended dosage.

So when visiting your doctor, request the "25(OH) D" test (also referred to as 25-hydroxyvitamin D test). Of two that are being ofered, this one ofers the best results for your overall health.

Most experts agree that the

majority of adults would need

~5,000 IU of vitamin D daily, with

a small percentage requiring

even higher amounts to achieve

that level of beneft.

Again, it is impossible to determine an all-inclusive daily requirement (above or below the

recommended daily allowance),

because dosage should be

efectively based on the results of

your personal blood test.

It is important to always check

with your doctor prior to taking a

dietary supplement. Do not stop

taking prescribed medications

without consulting your doctor.

TO UNDERSTAND YOUR VITAMIN D READINGS/RESULTS,

HERE ARE THE RANGES TO

CONSIDER, for all age categories:

• <20 ng/ml is considered

"Seriously Defcient"

• <50 ng/ml is considered

"Defcient"

• Between 50-70 ng/ml is

considered "Optimal"

• Between 70-100 ng/ml

"Benefcial" to preventing

serious health conditions

• >100 ng/ml is considered

"Excessive Dangerous"

++++++++++++++++++++++++++++++++

Resources:

1. European Society of Hypertension. "Vitamin D supplements can reduce blood pressure in patients with hypertension." ScienceDaily, 25 Apr. 2012. Web. 21 Apr. 2013.

2. http://dx.doi.org/10.1007/s12170-011-0186-0

3. http://dx.doi.org/10.1161/ HYPERTENSIONAHA.111.00659

4. Dr. Joseph Mercola. "Eliminate This Everyday Food and Watch Your High Blood Pressure Plunge". Mercola.com.

Natural Health Website. October 8, 2010. April 21, 2013.

http://articles.mercola.com/sites/articles/archive/2010/10/08/discover-the-secret-to-lowering-your-bloodpressure-in-15-minutes.aspx

5. Dr. Joseph Mercola. "How Much Vitamin D Do You Really Need to Take?". Mercola.com Natural Health Website.

October 10, 2009. April 21, 2013.

http://articles.mercola.com/sites/articles/archive/2009/10/10/Vitamin-D-Experts-Reveal-the-Truth.aspx

---

Grape Seed Extract

Grape seed extract, (GSE), is made from the seeds of red grapes, which are rich in vitamin E, and linoleic acid. GSE, as well as all parts of red grapes (juice, skin and the seeds) is one of the most powerful sources of the favonoid known as a proanthocyanidin, which is said to aid in reducing high blood pressure.

Research evidence has indicated that in a study including participants with metabolic syndrome who received 150 mg and 300 mg per day of GSE, lower blood pressure readings were achieved. Experts believe that the favor-able result in improved blood pressure was due to the proanthocyanidin in the grape seed extract, which has a natural arterial relaxing efect.

+++++++++++++++++++++++++++++++

85

Additional studies indicate that grape seed extract is benefcial to improving cardiovascular disease, such as hypertension, as well as a positive improvements in blood cholesterol levels, ultimately by supporting better blood fow.

Including red grapes as a part of a heart-healthy diet is the best way to naturally receive the benefts of the antioxidants and favonoids of this powerful fruit. Dietary GSE supplements are another alternative, however scientifc evidence only supports the use of red grape seed extract (as opposed to white grapes).

Resources:

1. http://dx.doi.org/10.1016/S0027-5107(02)00324-X

2. http://dx.doi.org/10.1016/j.jada.2011.05.015

3. Byron J. Richards, Board Certifed Clinical Nutritionist. Grape Seed Extract Lowers Blood Pressure. WellnessResources.com.Wellness Resources. Monday, February 04, 2013.May 24, 2013.

http://www.wellnessresources.com/health/articles/grape_seed_extract_lowers_blood_p

---

Flax Seeds

Flax seeds are high in fber and Omega-3 fatty acids, and are a good source of vitamin B1, as well. They also contain phytochemicals called lignans, which act as an antioxidant in killing of the harmful free radicals that can cause various diseases.

+++++++++++++++++++++++++++++++

Research studies support that faxseed may be benefcial for your heart health, and signifcantly aid in reducing high blood pressure levels for those with hypertension.

Flaxseed is available in two forms; whole or ground, and can be found at most all retail grocery and health food stores. Health experts suggest that ground faxseed is more easily digestible, therefore allowing your body to get the most benefts. Whole faxseed can be purchased and ground using a small cofee or spice grinder.

However, before purchasing faxseed, there are a pro's and con's to consider, in comparison.

Whole Flaxseed:

Pro: Longer shelf life (~6-12 months if stored properly) than ground faxseed Ground Flaxseed:

Pro: Convenient, and easily digested.

Whether you purchase whole and use freshly ground, or purchase pre-ground faxseed, it's important to consider the shelf life. Once ground, they are more prone to spoilage (due to oxidation), therefore have a shorter shelf life (~6-16 weeks) than whole faxseed.

It is best to store faxseed in an airtight container in a dark, cool place, preferably refrigerated. If using a glass container for storage, choosing a dark color helps reduce light exposure, extending freshness.

+++++++++++++++++++++++++++++++

Flaxseed oil has a sweet, nutty favor, and also ofers the same health benefts as ground faxseed. However the oil should be used only for favor-ing foods that have already been cooked. It is not recommended to use faxseed oil for cooking, and to always store in the refrigerator, as it is particularly perishable.

Since faxseed is high in fber, it is recommended that it should be taken with sufcient amounts of water or other fuids. As with any dietary supplement, always seek the advice of your physician before including it in your health plan.

Resources:

1.Faintuch J, Bortolotto LA, Marques PC *et al.* Systemic infammation and carotid diameter in obese patients: pilot comparative study with faxseed powder and cassava powder. Nutr Hosp. 2011 Jan-Feb;26(1):208-13. 2011.

2. n.a., "Flaxseeds: What's New and Benefcial about Flaxseeds", The World's Healthiest Foods, The George Mateljan Foundation, n.d, May 24, 2013,

http://www.whfoods.com/genpage.php?tname=foodspice&dbid=81#purchasequalities
3. Katherine Zeratsky, r.d., ld., "Does Ground Flaxseed Have More Health Benefts than Whole Flaxseed?". MayoClinic, Mayo Foundation for Medical Education and Research (MFMER), Jan. 19, 2013. May 24, 2013.

http://www.mayoclinic.com/health/faxseed/AN01258

++++++++++++++++++++++++++++++

88

Category 3: Reducing Body Fat

There is no doubt about the link between being

overweight and high blood pressure. In this section I will share with you the basics of how I lost 31

pounds of body fat in 90 days. If you want more in

depth information on the subject of fat loss I'll provide you with a resource that I highly recommend

at the end of this chapter. But in this section I want

to share with you the basics and enough for you to

get started on the right foot.

Have a Big Reason Why

This is a critical component to breaking any old habit and starting a new one. You must know your own internal 'reason why' that losing weight is so important for you to achieve. For me, it was the example that I wanted to set for my four kids. I did not want them to think that once you are out of shape that its all over. I wanted them to know that no matter what circumstance you fnd yourself in, you can always make better choices and over time completely change your life. This was going to be a real life lesson that I wanted for my kids...part of my legacy to them. Now I have to tell you...that is a BIG reason why and it keeps me motivated to this very day!

Follow A "Real Food" Diet

The recommended foods listed earlier in this book are all considered 'real foods' and will provide excellent nutritional value to your body. What do I mean by "real foods"? Basically it means only eating things that grew from the ground or had a parent. This means animal products, vegetables, nuts and seeds, and some fruit. By eating only real foods, many people notice +++++++++++++++++++++++++++++++

89

an immediate 7-10 pound drop in body weight as their body sheds itself of many of the toxins and excess water (from too much sodium) that they have been carrying around. To begin, just slowly start adding more "real foods"

into your diet each week. At the same time you will want to start eliminating the overly processed and manufactured bad foods from your diet.

Pre-cook Your Food

One of the things that really helped me stay on track was to pre-cook my food for the week. This meant that I was no longer scrambling to fnd something to eat when I got hungry, which lead to much better decision making on my part and a sense of control over my nutrition.

Limit Your Trips To Eat Out

Related to the previous tip, I would highly suggest giving up eating out for a while. Restaurants typically use way too much sodium or sodium like products in their pictures.

Drink Lots of Water

There is plenty of research that shows that thirst is often misinterpreted by the body as hunger. Often, drinking a full glass of water and waiting 10

minutes will take hunger pains away. In addition, being dehydrated by as little as 2% can cause headaches, fatigue, and slow your metabolism.

Remember, your biochemistry relies on water for it to work. Without plenty of water, your cells do not function at optimum levels and this makes losing fat very hard.

Get Plenty of Sleep

The nighttime cycle of rest and regeneration is often overlooked as part of a sensible fat loss plan. However, I want you to know that it is essential. As
+++++++++++++++++++++++++++++++

90

your body rests and repairs the cellular damage from a normal day's activities, your body is also releasing powerful fat fghting hormones…as long as you are getting deep, restful sleep.

Measure Your Carb Consumption

Without any doubt, the number one thing I recommend to friends and family who ask me how they can lose weight, is to drop their carbohydrate consumption down to under 100 grams of carbohydrates per day to start with. This will blunt the release of insulin into your system and help to keep fat burning going. If you go over 100 grams of carbohydrates and begin to inch up towards 150 grams of carbohydrates per day, you will begin to notice fat starting to be deposited around your middle again. The release of insulin in your body not only causes fat to be stored in your body, but studies also clearly show its link to high blood pressure. In fact, recent research shows that the more added sugar you have in your diet (which spikes insulin in your body) the higher risk you have for having hypertension.

Resources:

1. Mayo Clinic Staf. "Water: How much should you drink every day?" Nutrition and healthy eating. Mayo Clinic.

Mayo Foundation for Medical Education and Research. June 9, 2011. April 23, 2011.

http://www.mayoclinic.com/health/AboutThisSite/AM00057

2. Journal Of The American Medical Association. "Insufcient Sleep Associated With Overweight And Obesity."

ScienceDaily, 20 Jan. 2005. Web. 23 Apr. 2013.

3. "Increased Fructose Associates with Elevated Blood Pressure" PubMed.gov.

http://www.ncbi.nlm.nih.gov/pubmed/20595676

++++++++++++++++++++++++++++++

91

Category 4: Exercise

There are specifc kinds of exercises that can be

done at home, with no additional equipment other

than your body weight, which can dramatically improve your cardiovascular health. They also trigger

the release of benefcial hormones that will help

you burn fat. In this section I'll share with you the

type of exercises that I personally do that put me

in the best shape of my life and has kept me there.

All without fancy equipment.

Remember, the reason we are adding exercise to your health plan is to do the following:

1. Preserve muscle mass

2. Trigger release of fat burning hormones

3. Improve cardiovascular health

4. Increase metabolism

If you are very out of shape and have not done much, if any, physical exercise in the past several years, then the exercises show below will be the perfect way to get back into working out. All of these exercises can be done at home and with no additional equipment.

You will set up your workouts based on a seven-day schedule. This allows you to keep a consistent schedule and fts in perfectly with the overall Blood Pressure Solution program.

+++++++++++++++++++++++++++++++

92

This workout is designed to allow

anyone to start moving, and gain

the confdence and strength

needed to transition into more

advanced workouts when you are

ready.

The principle behind this exercise is

that by using your own body weight

you will create resistance and

begin to work your heart and cardiovascular system. The idea with

this workout is to work briskly and

complete each workout as fast as

you can. These workouts are meant

to take around 7-8 minutes each.

That's all…just 7-8 minutes per day

of exercise! You may be wondering

if exercising that little each day can

have much of an impact on your

health. Indeed it can if you keep the

intensity level high enough.

How do you ramp up the intensity of the workouts? The trick is to complete the work as fast as possible and make the exercise as intense as you can while still staying within the range of safety. The very best way to do this is to keep track of the time it takes you to complete the exercises below. Each time you perform them, try to beat your old time by a few seconds. If you continue to do this, you will essentially be working harder each time. This is QUICK NOTE ON TERMI-NOLOGY:

In the descriptions I use the

term 'round'. A round is simple one cycle through a set

of exercises. If I was to say

do two rounds of 10 pushups

and 10 air squats, then you

would complete the exercises

in this order:

Round 1:

10 pushups

10 air squats

Round 2:

10 pushups

10 air squats

++++++++++++++++++++++++++++++

93

the key to keeping intensity high. Ok, so let's dive into the Blood Pressure Solution workout. You can fnd the videos for these exercises on our site here.

Day One: (typically a Sunday)

this is a non-workout day, which allows your body to rest and recover.

Day Two:

- Warm Up: March in Place (4 minutes)

- 3 Rounds of:

* 3 Get Ups!

Get Ups! These are simply lying down on the ground on your back fully extended, and then getting up into a standing position. Simple yet efective!

Do this as quickly as possible.

++++++++++++++++++++++++++++++

94

* 10 Air Punches

Air Punches is simply standing with one foot in front of the other and then punching the air in front of you as if you were a boxer punching a bag.

Alternate between right and left arms.

Record your total time to complete this entire Day Two exercise program.

Next time, try to beat your old time just a bit.

Day Three:

This is a non-workout day, but I want you to take a 10-minute walk to keep your muscles moving. This is a slow, leisurely walk.

++++++++++++++++++++++++++++++

95

Day Four:

- Warm Up: March in Place (4 minutes)

- 3 Rounds of:

* 10 Wall Pushes

A Wall Push is simply walking up to a wall, keeping your feet about 2' away from the wall, then leaning into the wall with your outstretched hands.

Then you will do the same motion as if you were doing a push up, but in this case you are pushing against the wall.

++++++++++++++++++++++++++++++

96

* 10 Air Squats

An Air Squat mimics the movement you would do if you sat in a chair, but in this case there is no chair. You simply squat down as you would to sit in a chair, and then stand back up. Keep your feet pointing forward, and your back straight.

Record your total time to complete this entire Day Four exercise program.

Next time, try to beat your old time just a bit.

Day Five:

This is a non-workout day, but I want you to take a 10-minute walk to keep your muscles moving. This is a slow, leisurely walk.

+++++++++++++++++++++++++++++++

97

Day Six:

- Warm Up: March In place (4 minutes)

- As many rounds as possible in 8 minutes:

*10 Wall Pushes

*10 Air Squats

*10 Air Punches

Day Seven:

This is a non-workout day, but I want you to take a 10-minute walk to keep your muscles moving. This is a slow, leisurely walk.

That's it! While this may look like a very simple exercise plan, you will fnd that by sticking with this very straightforward program you will begin to feel better, have more energy, and even start feeling stronger. The key is to continually ramp up the intensity. If you fnd that you have mastered these exercises and can blaze through them, you can begin to add hand weights to the workout when you do the air squats and air punches. You can even get a weighted vest to wear that will quickly ramp up the intensity!

IMPORTANT NOTE:

Day Six is a little diferent because I am asking you to workout for a solid 8 minutes without stopping. You will keep going until 8 minutes is up. Keep track of your total number of repetitions during this session and that will be the number you try to beat next time you do Day Six.

+++++++++++++++++++++++++++++++

The best beneft however, is that you will be conditioning your heart and blood vessels in a safe and efective way that will help to lower your overall blood pressure readings. Don't think that this simple exercise program is too easy for you! Try it out and you'll see that it works your whole body and that you will actually appreciate the rest days that are built in!

Resources:

1. http://dx.doi.org/10.1155/2011/868305

3. http://dx.doi.org/10.1002/ajhb.21166.

Category 5: Stress Reduction

The reduction of stress plays a very important role

in lowering blood pressure. If you think about this

it makes sense. When you are stressed your heart

rate elevates, you tense up, and your biochemistry

changes. Each of these things contributes to your

blood pressure rising. In this section I'll show you

some extremely efective ways to lower your blood

pressure with nothing more than your breathing,

your mind, and a few simple techniques.

As discussed, we know that the primary things to consider in staying on the path to

wellness is to consistently follow a healthy diet and exercise routine,
++++++++++++++++++++++++++++++++

99

get the essential sleep your body needs to heal and rejuvenate, and avoid any consumption of alcohol, tobacco products, or other toxic addictions.

So in this chapter, we are going to focus primarily on the dangerous health efects of stress, and how mind-body interventions can play a role in reducing these efects. You will also learn a few simple techniques that you can incorporate into your daily health plan, taking just a matter of minutes, to help you manage your daily stresses.

To begin, we can easily agree that we all experience some form of stress on a regular basis, it's practically unavoidable, right? Who hasn't ever wished to for the ability to just crawl into an imaginary hole of avoidance, desperately hoping that the momentary crisis will just magically go away? So it's fairly easy to recognize the outward symptoms of stress, often manifested as avoidance, anxiety, anger, depression, headaches, insomnia… the list can go on. But have you ever considered what's simultaneously happening to you on the inside?

To briefy explain the natural biological process, your body responds to stress by releasing a food of hormones, which triggers an increase in your heart rate and the narrowing of your blood vessels, which then results in temporary spikes in your blood pressure levels.

In the heat of the moment, this short term elevation shouldn't put your body any immediate danger, however science has proven that the long-term efects of this physical reaction to stress can put you at risk for developing serious health conditions, among them being hypertension.

++++++++++++++++++++++++++++++++

100

While it has not been scientifcally proven that stress actually causes high blood pressure, studies do indicate that there is indeed a link between blood pressure and stress. During a three-month study, conducted by Dr.

Randy Zusman, an expert in treating hypertensive patients, and in conjunction with Boston's Benson-Henry Institute for Mind Body Medicine, patients who were being treated with hypertension medications began participating in relaxation training.

Although somewhat skeptical of the efect that meditative actions would result in any signifcant results, Zusman was pleased to fnd encouraging results in about 40-60 of the patients involved in the study.

"Their blood pressure dropped, and they dropped some of their medication.

It was striking. It was statistically signifcant, but more important it was clinically signifcant to these people," he says.

The doctor did further conclude that there is work involved in achieving these type of results. Learning to properly utilize the techniques, and becoming dedicated to following a daily meditation practice, is essential to achieving long-term results, as indicated by the study patients who succeed-ed in lowering their blood pressure.

So if you have been diagnosed with high blood pressure, or are concerned about it's development, it's time to do something about it. Seriously, by dedicating yourself to taking command of your health and actively committing yourself to making permanent lifestyle changes, you can fnd yourself on the path of least resistance, steadily progressing toward better health.

So how do you get the upper hand in your stress life? Realistically, it's your behavior (not the problem itself) that should be your frst consideration. It's imperative that you grasp this truth… while you can't eliminate everything
++++++++++++++++++++++++++++++++

101

that causes complications in your life; you can (and MUST) take control of your reactions to them when they occur.

The frst step you need to take in order to reduce your risk is to properly identifying each of the behaviors or circumstances that are the root cause your stress. Then you must learn to efectively manage your reactions to those triggers. This process is not difcult at all, but it is something that must become a habit, and incorporated into your daily routine.

Mind-Body Interventions

Research has shown that a large majority of Americans are using comple-mentary and alternative medicine treatments, commonly referred to as mind-body interventions. This might involve meditation, relaxation, and breathing techniques, biofeedback, autogenic training, acupuncture, and herbal remedies, for the purpose of treating many health conditions. Below are brief explanations for a few of these stress-relieving techniques that are worthy of consideration.

Meditation

Meditation is a practice that is often misunderstood, for a variety of reasons.

The most common assumption is that meditation is just a type of religious practice, however this isn't always the case. The intent for meditation is learning to control your thoughts, creating within yourself a state of inner awareness, calming your mind, and relieving tension.

As do many, you might consider meditation to be another "new age trend". So before you head for the hills, assuming that this is some super-

+++++++++++++++++++++++++++++++++

natural notion of being transported into some "Never-land of Ethereal Bliss", please trust that this is not what we are suggesting.

Simply put, meditation is merely an efective method of relaxing your mind, body, and spirit, which can be benefcial to anyone. We recommend meditation by this defnition, because it has been scientifcally proven to play a role in reducing stress, thereby reducing the associated health risks.

There are actually numerous types of meditational practices, which can range from a simple state of "daydreaming" to one that maintains a highly spiritual or religious focus. The techniques can vary by culture, and many are distinctive to each individual. But regardless of the specifc technique, the basic premise of practicing any form of meditation is to focus your mind in a positive direction, and improve your sense of well-being.

So if you have never experienced meditation, have an open mind, and give it a try. Here are a few of the traditional methods:

• Guided Meditation: This option can be done by listening to a recorded message, or having someone speak/read a guided meditation to you. This script may include instructions such as, "sit comfortably with your eyes closed... take deep, slow breaths… picture yourself in a specifc surrounding", *etc.* The process of allowing your mind to follow along with the soothing presentation of the scripted message, is for the purpose of reaching a state of deep relaxation, leaving your conscious state of mind at rest, releasing your mind to subconsciously envision freeing your mind of the negative, and replacing it with positive and encouraging thoughts.

++++++++++++++++++++++++++++++

103

• Zen Meditation: This type involves the practice of sitting in various positions, relaxing your mind and body. The idea is to rid your mind of all thoughts and images, focusing only on the present, as your breathing and heart rate slow down. This is said to allow your mind to escape from the past and future, and enjoy the peace of the moment.

• Mindfulness Meditation: This simple technique involves teaching your mind to be aware of the actions and situations that surround your life. The goal is the create a better sense of relaxation and acceptance with regard to the things we cannot change, and take control of those that we can change. With practical purposes, your concentration is centered deliberately on the causes of your stress (whether diet, exercise, specifc health issues, etc.), and maintaining the discipline necessary to improve those things according to your ability.

• Imagery meditation: This simple technique is one that can be done either in a group setting, or individually. The idea is that there is an "imagined scene", to which you build upon by adding scenes, creating an imaginary mental encounter. Some fnd it quite relaxing not only to explore their own imagination, but to also refect on the focus of the experience.

If you prefer something a little less conventional, here are a few meditative activities that you might want to consider:

• "Be Still and Silent": Find a quiet, comfortable place and spend ~15

minutes, eyes closed, concentrating on a singular positive thought or goal, efectively clearing your head of everything that negatively distracts you.

++++++++++++++++++++++++++++++

104

• "Process Proactively": If your racing mind is particularly challenged, spend a few minutes writing down the things that are scrambling your brainwaves, and process ways to prioritize and tackle them one at a time.

• "Get Moving": Put on some soothing music, and go for a walk (or run/

jog/bike ride, do some yoga/stretching exercises. Spend that time focused on calming your nerves by working out the things in your mind that might be causing your frustration.

However, regardless of what form of meditation you choose to participate in, your primary purpose is to clear your mind and release stress.

Breathing Exercises

"Just take a deep breath…" is the advice often given to those experiencing moments of stress and anxiety. But does this really work? The answer is, yes it does, when done properly. Breathing exercises have been used for thou-sands of years as a way of calming your nerves and clearing your mind.

The most common type is referred to as "diaphragmatic breathing" (deep abdominal breathing). It is said that this technique can be used efectively to lessen anyone's tension; leaving you feeling relaxed as you control your internal rhythm. For those who are interested in using this technique for the purpose of lowering blood pressure, it ofers excellent results when you are committed to practicing this method twice per day. Here are the basic steps:

+++++++++++++++++++++++++++++++++

105

• Place one hand on your chest, the other on your abdomen. Inhale deeply, checking to ensure that the hand on your abdomen raises higher than that on your chest, to allow enough air into your lungs.

• Calmly exhale, and begin inhaling, taking in a slow deep breath, and then hold it (but don't force it). To maintain control of your breath, count up to 7.

• At the count of 8, begin to exhale slowly, until all of the air is released.

Then contract your diaphragm muscles gently, and relax.

• As when inhaling, be mindful of exhaling deeply and completely, but without forcing yourself.

• Repeat this process 4 or 5 times. You should do 5 or 6 deep breaths, maintaining 5-6 breaths per minute.

A few practical tips when practicing breathing exercises...

• Practice early in the morning, (or late in the evening) when your mind and body are relatively at ease, and the air is pure.

• To achieve the best results, drink water approximately 30 minutes prior to beginning your exercises, and avoid practicing after consuming a meal.

• Surround yourself in an area that allows you to focus your attention strictly to the exercise, free of distraction.

• Keep in mind the importance of making your breathing smooth and efortless. Start out slowly and take it easy as to avoid forcing yourself during your breathing exercises.

++++++++++++++++++++++++++++++++

106

• As with anything, do not participate in the exercises if you are not feeling well, and always consult your physician prior to making changes in your diet and exercise routine.

Biofeedback and Autogenic Training

Two stress relieving techniques, which work well individually or in combination, are biofeedback and autogenic training.

• Biofeedback is a non-invasive technique which involves being connected to a machine that essentially trains you to do things such as consciously tightening or relaxing muscles, changing your breathing patterns, which can slow your heart rate. Based on the feedback you receive (via lights and sounds from the machine), you learn to be able to manage your stress by efectively controlling your muscle move-ments and breathing patterns.

• Autogenic Training is a type of self-hypnosis. This technique essentially learning how to reduce your tension by giving yourself silent instructions, such as "my head is clear and calm", "my body is completely still and relaxed". While you can become very relaxed, you will still be aware of what's going on around you.

Much like meditation, these techniques used alone or in conjunction with one another, allow you the freedom to control your thoughts and manage your stress in a safe and efective way.

+++++++++++++++++++++++++++++++

107

Audio (Binaural Beats)

Your brainwaves and state of consciousness can be directly afected by certain auditory frequencies, varying from a state of high alert to one of deep sleep. At certain frequencies, the use of this auditory brain stimulation is said to induce a sense of calm and relaxation.

The method of using binaural beats works by introducing 2 specifc auditory tones, with a separate frequency per ear, when heard through headphones.

Your brainwaves then perceive the tonal variance, and accommodate by producing a unifying third tone, in order to naturally follow along with the beat.

To better explain, for example, if 200Hz were being played in your left ear, and 207Hz in your right ear, your brain perceives a tone of 7Hz. It has been proven that by using this technique consistently, you allow your brainwaves to synchronize, which improves your thought processes.

Another great beneft of binaural beats (or tones), is that they cause your brain to start matching the frequency of the tone your brain perceives. In the previous example where your brain would perceive a tone of 7Hz, your brainwaves would quickly start matching this frequency. The beneft to this is that certain brainwave frequencies have been identifed that relate to certain specifc relaxation states. For instance, brainwave frequencies of 4-7

Hz have been identifed with deep meditative states, exactly what you need when you want to relax.

++++++++++++++++++++++++++++++++

108

Brainwave Classifcation Chart

Frequency

Range

Name Usually associated with:

100 to 200 Hz Lambda waves

Wholeness and integration, as well as with

mystical experiences and out of body

experiences (very high frequency brainwaves)

30 to 100 Hz

Gamma and Hyper-Gamma

waves

Higher mental activity; perception, problem

solving, fear, and consciousness

13 to 30 Hz Beta waves

Active, busy or anxious thinking and active

concentration, arousal, cognition, and/or

paranoia

8 to 12 Hz Alpha waves

Relaxation (while awake), pre-sleep and

pre-wake drowsiness, REM sleep, dreams

4 to 8 Hz Theta waves Deep meditation/relaxation, NREM sleep

0.5 to 4 Hz Delta waves

Deep dreamless sleep, loss of body

awareness

< 0.5 Hz Epsilon waves

Strongly related to Lambda (highest

frequency waves). The same states of

consciousness are associated with both

Lambda and Epsilon waves.

While binaural beats have been proven to afect each listener in a mental and physical
way, each individual hears the third "imaginary" tone diferently.

++++++++++++++++++++++++++++++++

There is some level of caution to consider for certain individuals and circumstances. The use of binaural beats is not recommended for those who are prone to seizures, children, or while operating any type of machinery. As with any health condition, it is important to consult your physician prior to using this technique.

Acupuncture

Acupuncture is a practice used both in traditional Chinese medicine, as well many practitioners of Western medicine. Though there is a variance in the purpose of practicing this alternative therapy, acupuncture has been shown to provide many health benefts. The technique involves stimulating the nerves in specifc places of the body, using very fne needles to puncture the skin.

During this process, your body naturally releases certain chemicals and hormones in your body, in order to allow the body to correct it's imbalances.

This procedure can also be accompanied the use of electric stimulation, transmitting low-frequency currents through the needles.

By correcting the root problems associated with hypertension, such as the condition of your nervous system, blood vessels, and kidneys, either method of acupuncture is said to have a positive efect in lowering blood pressure.

Acupuncture can be a safe, low-risk option for treating the symptoms associated with high blood pressure, but should be done only by a professionally licensed practitioner. Please do not stop taking any prescribed medications prior to seeking the advice of your physician.

+++++++++++++++++++++++++++++++

110

Oolong Tea

Tea, arguably one of the most popular beverages worldwide, serves a higher purpose than just liquid refreshment. Sipping a hot cup of Oolong tea is a great way to relax and unwind, and there's even an added bonus. Studies have long shown that tea contains powerful antioxidants, varying in degree by type, that provide a range of health benefts.

Oolong tea, (which is a diferent type than green tea or black tea), has been proven efective in promoting weight loss and heart health, and lowering blood pressure, just to name a few. There has been much research over the years regarding the health benefts of drinking tea, but scientists in Taiwan have completed what they believe is to be the frst study that provides clear evidence indicating that regular consumption of tea can reduce the risk of hypertension.

When the participants had met the criteria needed, researchers were somewhat surprised to fnd that the study participants considered to be habitual tea drinkers, tended to exhibit behaviors that put them at a higher risk level for hypertension, than those considered to be non-habitual tea drinkers. In addition to being generally more obese, the habitual tea drinkers also had higher tendencies to maintaining a poor dietary routine (high in sodium, and low in vegetables), as well as exhibiting more addictive behaviors (smoking and alcohol) in comparison to the non-tea drinkers.

However, the fndings reported that despite these risk factors, the blood pressure readings for those who drank tea regularly were still lower than those of the non-tea drinkers. The study authors found that the most exciting results in their fndings what the signifcant decrease in numbers of those who ultimately developed hypertension over the course of the study.

+++++++++++++++++++++++++++++++++

111

The researchers concluded that, "Compared with non-habitual tea drinkers, the risk of developing hypertension decreased by 46% for those who drank 120 to 599 milliliters per day, and was further reduced by 65% for those who drank 600 milliliters per day or more…". So evidence indicates that by regularly consuming oolong tea, you are increasing your ability to naturally lower your blood pressure, and reduce your risk of hypertension.

So cold or hot, oolong tea is a refreshing way to sit back and relax, and relieve some stress.

Sleep

Just like many of us reaching the end of a long day, you're likely desperate to bring that day to and end, and just go to sleep. But how often do you fnd yourself tossing and turning, in a constant struggle to get some shut-eye?

Poor sleep not only causes stress and understandable fatigue, but it can lead to some

serious health complications that should not be ignored, particularly if you have high blood pressure.

There have been many studies showing that insomnia, or a lack of sufcient sleep, can be directly related to having high blood pressure. But if you are among the millions who been diagnosed with hypertension, there is even more bad news. Researchers are now discovering that you are likely to double your risk of developing a resistance case of hypertension if you aren't getting the rest you need.

++++++++++++++++++++++++++++++++

112

So what does this mean? Bottom line-you could be facing the possibility of being prescribed at least three hypertension medications, which unfortunately may prove to be inefective in maintaining healthy blood pressure readings. Additionally, you're facing the challenge of a greater risk of developing any number of other associated diseases, which isn't encouraging.

Biologically, when we are under stress, our bodies react by releasing chemicals into our system in an efort to keep everything functioning properly. Not only are our minds and bodies working overtime, so are our major organs. Without proper diet and exercise, as well as adequate sleep, our systems will wear down and start to malfunction, causing all sorts of problems. Let's take a look at how a lack of sleep plays a role in this malfunctioning process.

For illustration purposes, let's say you fnd that over the years, you've put on a few unwanted pounds. As you've aged, and your metabolism is beginning to slow down, your weight is steadily increasing. Without having made any positive improvements in your diet and exercise routine, you've reached the point of being considered overweight, or ofcially obese. By now, in doing absolutely nothing, you've already placed yourself at a higher risk of developing any number of diseases.

Since we're focusing on your resting period, let's start with sleep apnea, for example. This is a condition in which you wake up gasping for air, several times during the course of the night, obviously causing disruption to your sleep patterns. Now let's say that this lack of quality sleep then turns into eating "fast food" because you're too tired to have to prepare anything ++++++++++++++++++++++++++++++++

113

healthy. As the pounds are adding up, so is your risk for developing hypertension, diabetes, and kidney problems (assuming you don't have it already).

Without any major modifcations in your lifestyle, you'll still fnd that you're not getting enough rest, because the stress of dealing with these conditions is keeping you up all night!

This frustrating cycle of "cause and efect" symptoms are clear indicators that your biological system is all out of whack. If you're not taking these symptoms seriously, you're just pushing yourself closer toward coronary heart disease, stroke, or worse… death.

"Not getting enough sleep" can lead to some pretty scary stuf, if you're not careful. But by making some adjustments in your sleeping habits, in addition to other necessary lifestyle changes, you can get one step closer to lowering your blood pressure, and improving your health.

Tips for improving your blood pressure readings by getting some quality Zzzz's:

• Sleep According to Schedule: go to bed and wake up at the same time, every single day. This consistency promotes better sleep at night.

• Stay Calm: if you fnd yourself tossing and turning, get up and do something relaxing. Stressing about getting to sleep is counterproduc-tive.

• Don't Go to Bed Hungry…or Full: avoid the distraction of gastrointestinal discomfort.

++++++++++++++++++++++++++++++++

114

• Limit Your Liquids: try to prevent those late night trips to the rest-room. Avoid alcohol, nicotine, and cafeine, each of which has stimulating efects.

• Create a Bedtime Ritual: take a shower, listen to soothing music, read a book, meditate… make relaxing a nightly habit to signal your body that it's time to go to sleep

• Create a Comfort Zone: create an environment that is comfortable for sleeping… not too hot, not too cold… not too bright, but just right.

Be sure that when you are going to sleep, your bed is comfy cozy.

• Try a Catnap: avoid taking a long nap during the day, which inter-rupts your normal sleep cycle. If you feel that you need to rest during the day, keep it quick. Enjoy an afternoon nap, but only for ~10-30

minutes.

• Get Physical: maintain a regular exercise schedule, planning your physical activity well before bedtime, to avoid being too energized to sleep.

• Get a Grip: prioritize and organize to manage your daily stressors. Be intentional about creating time for yourself to unwind, using whatever relaxation techniques necessary to calm your mind, and relieve your stress.

Pick up the Phone: if your inability to sleep is causing disruption that is afecting your health, call your doctor. Seek the advice of a professional to diagnose and treat any potential disorders that may be keeping you up at night.

+++++++++++++++++++++++++++++++

115

So in the end, when facing the challenges of managing hypertension, and reducing your risk of developing other associated diseases, it's important to have a plan. You must be prepared to make whatever lifestyle changes necessary will allow you to improve your health.

In addition to a proper diet and exercise routine, it's imperative to give equal consideration to spending time relaxing. Your body requires rest in order to rejuvenate and to function properly. As with anything, there isn't a "one-size-fts-all" method of relaxation. So feel free to try diferent techniques and see what suits you.

Either way, your end goal is always that of relieving your mind of anxiety.

Managing your stress, which can have an immediate afect on your blood pressure, will allow you to gain a better sense of well-being. There's nothing more peaceful than the feeling of being in control of living a happy, healthy life.

Resources:

1. Allison Aubrey, "To Lower Blood Pressure, Open Up and Say 'Om', NPR.org, http://www.npr.org/2008/08/21/93796200/to-lower-bloodpressure-open-up-and-say-om, April 17, 2013

2. http://dx.doi.org/10.1038/ajh.2007.65

3. http://dx.doi.org/10.1212/01.wnl.0000314667.16386.5e

4. Mayo Clinic Staf. "Stress and high blood pressure: What's the Connection?", MayoClinic.com, Mayo Foundation for Medical Education and Research (MFMER),

http://www.mayoclinic.com/health/stress-and-highblood-pressure/HI00092, Apr. 16, 2013

++++++++++++++++++++++++++++++

116

5. Kiks, "Basic Meditation Techniques", ProjectMeditation.org, http://www.project-meditation.org/a_mt4/basic_meditation_techniques.html April 16, 2013

6. Mary Jones, "Guided Meditation", ProjectMeditation.org, http://www.project-meditation.org/mt/guided_meditation.html , April 16, 2013

7. Kundan Pandey. Deep Breathing Exercises to Lower Blood Pressure. buzzle.com.2/29/2012. April 17, 2013

8. n.a. "The Complete Guide to Binaural Beats". binauralbrains.com. n.d., http://binauralbrains.com/ April 17, 2013

9. Mayo Clinic Staf. "Acupuncture", MayoClinic.com, Mayo Foundation for Medical Education and Research (MFMER), http://www.mayoclinic.com/health/acupuncture/MY00946, April 17, 2013

10. Robin Springer L.Ac., MS, CMT. "Can Acupuncture Help Lower High Blood Pressure?", Essential Wellness, Sept.

11, 2012, http://essentialwellnesssf.com/2012/09/can-acupuncture-help-lower-highblood-pressure/, April 17, 2013

11. Editorial Team, "Acupuncture to lower blood Pressure", Onlymyhealth.com, Feb. 6, 2013, April 17, 2013

12. n.a. "Study: Daily Tea Consumption Reduces Risk of Hypertension". Acupuncture Today.

October, 2004, Volume 05, Issue 10. Web.

http://healthsolutionssource.com/StudyDailyTeaConsumption.pdf, April 17, 2013

13. Maureen Salamon, "Poor Sleep May Make High Blood Pressure Worse". HealthDay. U.S. News & World Report, September 21, 2012. Web. April 17, 2013

14. n.a. "Sleeping Longer At Night Could Improve Blood Pressure Levels: Study", HufngtonPost.com. Dec. 10, 2012. April 17, 2013. http://www.hufngtonpost.com/2012/12/10/sleep-blood-pressure-duration-bedtime-hypertension_n_2238135.html

15. Mayo Clinic Staf. Adult Health. "Sleep Tips: 7 steps to better sleep", MayoClinic.com, Mayo Foundation for Medical Education and Research (MFMER), http://www.mayoclinic.com/health/sleep/HQ01387, April 17, 2013

16. Dr. Natural. "Autogenic Training and Biofeedback". Natural Health.com. March 23, 2009. April 17, 2013.

http://natural-health.most-efective-solution.com/2009/03/autogenic-training-and-biofeedback/

+++++++++++++++++++++++++++++++

Category 6: Eliminating Toxins

As you know, the things we put into our body can

either help us or harm us. Two of the major

ofenders when it comes to high blood pressure

are smoking and alcohol use. In this section we'll

take a close-up look at these two substances to

understand how they negatively impact blood

pressure.

Smoking and High Blood Pressure

One of the lesser-known impacts of smoking is that it raises your blood pressure. With each inhalation, the toxic nicotine constricts your arteries.

This constriction reduces the area inside your arteries, permitting less room for blood to fow through, thereby raising blood pressure. Having watched several family members struggle with smoking addiction, I'm sensitive to those that want to quit but are having trouble. Just imagine with me for a moment....

If you quit smoking right now... Twenty minutes after you stop smoking, your heart rate slows down to a calm, steady beat, lowering your blood pressure.

Eight to twelve hours later, the dangerous levels of carbon monoxide in your blood have now dropped to a normal level. You may start to feel relief from any fu-like symptoms-from everyday fatigue to headaches, sleepi-ness, and nausea, all of which could have resulted from the efects of carbon monoxide.

+++++++++++++++++++++++++++++++

Two days later, your heart attack risk is lower and continues to decline over the next three months. You'll suddenly notice you don't need as much salt (thanks to a return in the sensitivity of your taste buds) – and the air smells fresh (now that your sense of smell has returned). Three days later you might feel like going for a jog – because your energy is going to skyrocket.

After the frst month, you have fewer instances of that annoying, hacking smoker's cough because your bronchial tubes are on the mend. Whenever your bronchial tubes are irritated, they produce excess mucus. So eliminate the cigarettes, and you can say goodbye to the nagging feeling of having to constantly clear your throat. A few months later, you'll be taking the stairs without gasping for a breath. As you get your body moving, your circulation will naturally improve, recovering from the efects of constricted blood vessels. Just one cigarette reduces the blood fow throughout your body for an hour.

The health improvements continue long after you quit smoking. Your gift at the frst anniversary of quitting is that your risk of coronary heart disease becomes half that of what you risked as a smoker.

HERE'S ANOTHER BENEFIT:

You'll keep aging signs at bay. The mouth suction that you use to puf on the cigarette is terrible for producing or deepening wrinkles.

When you stop smoking, you give those facial muscles a well-deserved rest.

+++++++++++++++++++++++++++++++++

119

Make it to your ffth year smoke-free, and your risk of stroke is the same as a non-smoker. That's really amazing! In ten years, your lungs become stronger, and your chances of dying from lung cancer are only half as great as if you continued to smoke.

Alcohol Consumption

If you consume more than 2 drinks per day (for men), or one drink per day (for women) then you are putting yourself at a much greater risk for high blood pressure.

Alcohol consumption impacts your health on many fronts. Two critical health conditions involved, with regard to hypertension are: OTHER RISKS DECREASE WHEN YOU END YOUR SMOKING

HABITS. Here are a few more to consider:

• Cancer

• Cardiovascular Disease

• Impotence

• Infertility

• Macular Degeneration

• Periodontal Disease

• Ulcers

+++++++++++++++++++++++++++++++

120

Weight gain

Due to the high sugar content in most alcoholic beverages your body will respond by fooding your bloodstream with insulin in order to marshal the sugar out of your bloodstream and into your cells. This sounds great, but the unfortunate side efect is that when insulin levels are high, all fat burning stops dead in its tracks. Think about that the next time you are drinking and also eating the chips, pretzels, and other foods that typically come along with alcohol consumption. The impact this has on your blood pressure has to do with the weight gain that alcohol can cause. More external pressure on your arteries means the pressure within those arteries is kept higher.

Overworking the liver

The second impact that alcohol has on your blood pressure has to do with the workload alcohol consumption puts on your liver. When the body detects alcohol in your system it treats it much like it would any toxin. It begins an all-hands-on-deck process to get it out of your body as fast as possible.

However, this is not as easy as it sounds. Alcohol must be broken down in your liver through a process called oxidation. Once the initial stages of oxidation occur about 10% of the remaining byproducts are eliminated from your body through your breath or your urine. The remaining 90% of the alcohol byproducts are further broken down in the liver and turned into acetic acid.

The problem this causes in relation to high blood pressure is that this process of breaking down alcohol takes a very long time and keeps your liver very busy trying to eliminate this toxin (alcohol) from your body. In fact, it takes a full hour for your body to eliminate the alcohol from just a 12-ounce beer. Imagine the length of time it would take to eliminate beverages with much higher alcohol content.

+++++++++++++++++++++++++++++++++

121

This is where it gets tricky. While your liver is busy using its resources to get rid of the alcohol, it has to neglect a few very important functions that are important to regulating blood pressure. There are two hormones, renin and angiotensin, that are essential to keeping your blood pressure within normal ranges. However, when your liver is overburdened with the high priority task of removing alcohol from your body, the production of these two important hormones is neglected.

Resources:

1. http://dx.doi.org/10.1161/ http://dx.doi.org/10.1161/ 01.HYP.37.2.187

2. http://dx.doi.org/10.1161/01.HYP.17.6.787

+++++++++++++++++++++++++++++++++

122

CHAPTER 7

The Blood Pressure Solution

Implementation Plan

Now it's time to show you how to take everything

you have learned about naturally lowering your

blood pressure and use it to create a personalized

plan that is right for you. This book has given you

a wealth of information about how to naturally

lower your blood pressure.

However, from this point forward I want you to

think of this book as a reference guide, rather than

a list of things you MUST do right now. It is here for you when you need it.

When you want to try something new, just pick up this guide and read about the next supplement, exercise, meditation technique, or food that you want to include in your new healthy lifestyle.

In fact, there is so much information given that a common response is to feel a bit overwhelmed. However, that needn't be the case. In fact, I want to share with you a very important tip…

+++++++++++++++++++++++++++++++

123

So relax! I am going to show you my top recommendations for your frst 30

days. This streamlined guide will make it very easy for you to plan and implement the next four weeks of meals, exercises, supplements, and relaxation strategies.

The goal is to build a daily plan for you that is easy to follow and gives you a framework for monitoring your results so that you can see your progress week to week.

THE TOP RECOMMENDATIONS that I have for quickly lowering

your blood pressure using the strategies in this book will fall into the following main categories:

• The Power of Measurements

• Your Daily Diet

• Exercise Explained

• Relax A Little

• Super Supplements

IMPORTANT TIP:

No one can implement everything in this book on day one!

+++++++++++++++++++++++++++++++

124

We will be using a common feedback mechanism to make sure you are continually moving toward normal blood pressure ranges. This tool is simply the three step process of Implementing - Monitoring - Adjusting.

This simple framework will be implemented on a seven day weekly schedule. This will create a predictable pattern for you and allows any changes you made to your diet, exercise, or supplements to show their efect by the time you take new measurements at the end of the week.

The Power of Measurements

It has long been known that if you want to improve some aspect of a person's performance, you simply begin measuring their results. The same idea applies to your health. The very act of measuring your blood pressure, weight, and body fat percentage will help you become more aware of what you are eating. In addition, the data from each measurement will give us valuable data points so that we can monitor the impact of your new choices.

If your measurements are not improving, then we know that we need to make adjustments. If they are improving, we know we are on the right track.

Your Daily Diet

The biggest leverage point we have to attack high blood pressure is your diet. By helping you transition to a lower carb, higher fat, medium protein diet that removes most processed sodium from your diet, you will begin to feel better within days and your blood pressure will begin to come down.

The included meal plan will help you tremendously to set up and plan your meals and grocery purchases.

+++++++++++++++++++++++++++++++

125

Exercise Explained

Having a strong cardiovascular system is one of the smartest things you can do to help naturally lower your blood pressure. We will use short, but intense, exercises to stimulate your cardiovascular system and help improve its capacity. In addition, the type of exercise you will be doing has been show to release certain very benefcial hormones that help with fat loss and also muscle retention.

Relax A Little

We all live in a more stressful time now than our ancestors did, so we will plan to incorporate two planned relaxation sessions per day for you. This is crucial and I can tell you from my own experience was one of the best things I did to help control my blood pressure. These times of slowing down for a few minutes each day really do have a big impact on my overall stress level, which we know contributes directly to your blood pressure readings.

Super Supplements

As much as we would all like to believe that our modern food supply can give us all the nutrition we need, the sad fact is that due to the modern processing of much of our food supply, many of the benefcial nutrients have been removed. To overcome this modern dilemma, we must make sure our bodies get the expected nutrients needed in order to operate efciently.

For this reason, many of us will need to supplement our diet with external sources. The supplements that I will list in this section are my top choices and support the process of naturally lowering your blood pressure.

++++++++++++++++++++++++++++++++

126

How To Create Your Personalized Plan

Now that you understand my top recommendations for lowering your blood pressure naturally, you can see how easy it will be to build out a seven-day schedule. All it takes is just flling in the information for each of the 5 major categories you will be working on each day.

Here is how to create your own personalized plan for a single day of the week. You will repeat this process for each of the seven days to create your weekly plan. In the description below, I include a lot of additional commen-tary for the sake of explaining this process. In your actual daily and weekly plans you can just list the measurement, food item, exercise, relaxation technique or supplement.

1. Take Your Measurements

Each Sunday I want you to take three measurements. First, I want you to record your body weight. As you know, losing weight is a very efective way to drop your blood pressure. Next, I want you to record your body fat percentage. This is also an indicator of obesity and will help us see the progress you are making. To calculate your body fat percentage, just type in your body weight and a few simple measurements into the tool in the BloodPressureSolution.com Member's Area, and it will calculate it for you.

With these three measurements, you will be able to clearly see any progress or regression you make each week, and clearly see if/when any adjustments are needed.

2. Assemble Your Meal Plan

To create your ideal diet I want you to use the included meal plans that came as part of your purchase. Simple choose the breakfast, lunch, and dinner options from the included meal plans. Each of these recipes has been created to be very high in foods that will naturally lower your blood pressure. In addition to adding in these benefcial foods, one of the most important things you can do is to reduce your sodium intake.

3. Plan Your Exercise

Since exercise has been shown to greatly help to lower blood pressure naturally, you will refer to chapter 5 of this book and follow the exercise plan that was outlined there day by day. The exercise plan in that chapter steps you through all seven days of the week, and tells you exactly what to do. This exercise plan was created to trigger the release of fat burning hormones and other benefcial hormones that will aid in fat loss, and is proven highly efective. It only takes 7-8 minutes a day as well.

4. Take Time To Relax

Each day I want you to set aside two 10-minute periods of time when you will utilize one of the relaxation methods presented in this book. I suggest taking 10 minutes in the morning shortly after you get up, and also one just prior to going to bed in the evening. Pick two of the relaxation methods presented in the chapter on Relaxation. You don't have to be a hard-core meditator to do this. Some of my best and most relaxing times were simply laying down, listening to calming music and doing deep breathing.

It is amazing how rejuvenating these simple actions can be on both your mental outlook and also your internal health!

5. Supercharging Your Results With Supplements

Far and away the best supplements for naturally lowering your blood pressure are listed below. I use a special combination of these supplements daily and so does my dad, who you heard about when you purchased this program. I always recommend getting as much of the vitamins and recommended minerals from your daily diet as possible, however that is not always possible. That is why supplementation is so important.

Now without further ado…let's get to these Super Supplements!

Super Supplement #1: Omega-3s

Omega-3s are derived from the fatty oil of cold-water fsh such as herring, cod, mackerel, and salmon. The fatty acids that make up Omega-3s (EPA and DHA) have been proven to help lower infammation in the body. Research data has shown that Omega-3s have made an impact on lowering blood pressure in study participants. Click Here for a FREE TRIAL of my favorite Omega 3 supplement.

Super Supplement #2: Magnesium

Magnesium is a very important mineral in your body that is necessary for over 300 biomechanical processes within your body to occur. Without proper levels of magnesium, your body simply cannot function optimally.

In addition magnesium seems to help regulate blood pressure in your body.

Super Supplement #3: Potassium

While high levels of sodium can increase your blood pressure, high levels of potassium seem to act the opposite way and reduce your risk of high blood pressure. "High potassium levels may act as a diuretic, causing sodium to
+++++++++++++++++++++++++++++++

129

be excreted," Paul Whelton, MD says. "Or potassium may dilate and relax the muscles in blood vessel walls." Interestingly, this mineral has also been found to reduce the risk of stroke, yet "most Americans get only half their recommended allowance [4,700 milligrams a day]," says Whelton.

Super Supplement #4: Hawthorne

Hawthorn is an herb that has been used for centuries to help lower blood pressure and has the support of many top doctors. According to Dr. James Meschino, recognized as a leading expert in nutrition, anti-aging, ftness and wellness, "Scientifc and clinical investigations have shown that active constituents in hawthorn extract can reduce high blood pressure via their infuence on the angiotensin system, by acting as calcium channel blockers and by improving endothelial function.

Super Supplement #5: Grape Seed Extract

Two new studies suggest grape seed extract may beneft hypertension, cholesterol and glycemic response. The trials, conducted by University of California Davis research scientists, used grape seed extracts from polyphe-nols and the results were published in the Journal of Pharmacy and Nutrition Sciences and Functional Foods in Health and Disease. This study was undertaken to determine whether a grape seed extract (GSE) which is a nutraceutical containing vasodilator phenolic compounds lowers blood pressure in subjects with prehypertension.

Super Supplement #6: D3

Scientifc studies have concluded that vitamin D defciency has been associated with a group of health problems, including insulin resistance, obesity, and hypertension. In addition to it's involvement in regulating your
++++++++++++++++++++++++++++++++

130

immune system, (relevant due to its ability to decrease infammation), vitamin D has also been shown to reduce systolic blood pressure, and is a requirement for statins (drugs prescribed to lower cholesterol levels) to work efectively, as well.

Super Supplement #7: CoEnzyme Q10

CoEnzyme Q10 is a powerful vitamin-like substance that several studies show as being benefcial to lowering blood pressure.

Super Supplement #8: Nitrates

Nitrates are powerful substances within certain foods that, when consumed, are converted to nitric oxide within our bodies. Nitric oxide has the efect of relaxing and dilating blood vessels in your body, which increases blood fow and volume within the blood vessel itself. This has the efect of lowering blood pressure, sometimes quite dramatically. Several studies have shown that beetroot juice, when consumed daily, can signifcantly reduce blood pressure levels in only 24 hrs. Scientists believe that this is a result of the nitrates, which naturally occur in foods such as beetroot juice.